Pediatrics

Editors

KRISTYN S. LOWERY
BRIAN R. WINGROVE
GENEVIEVE A.N. DELROSARIO

PHYSICIAN ASSISTANT CLINICS

www.physicianassistant.theclinics.com

Consulting Editor
JAMES A. VAN RHEE

October 2016 • Volume 1 • Number 4

ELSEVIER

1600 John F. Kennedy Boulevard • Suite 1800 • Philadelphia, Pennsylvania, 19103-2899

http://www.theclinics.com

PHYSICIAN ASSISTANT CLINICS Volume 1, Number 4
October 2016 ISSN 2405-7991, ISBN-13: 978-0-323-46329-4

Editor: Jessica McCool
Developmental Editor: Casey Jackson

Physician Assistant Clinics (ISSN: 2405–7991) is published quarterly by Elsevier Inc., 360 Park Avenue South, New York, NY 10010-1710. Months of issue are January, April, July, and October. Periodicals postage paid at New York, NY and additional mailing offices. Subscription prices are $150.00 per year (US individuals), $195.00 (US institutions), $100.00 (US students), $150.00 (Canadian individuals), $245.00 (Canadian institutions), $100.00 (Canadian students), $150.00 (international individuals), $245.00 (international institutions), and $100.00 (international students). Foreign air speed delivery is included in all *Clinics* subscription prices. All prices are subject to change without notice. POSTMASTER: Send address changes to *Physician Assistant Clinics*, Elsevier Periodicals Customer Service, 11830 Westline Industrial Drive, St. Louis, MO 63146. Customer Service Health Sciences Division, Subscription Customer Service, 3251 Riverport Lane, Maryland Heights, MO 63043. **Customer Service: 1-800-654-2452 (U.S. and Canada); 314-447-8871 (outside U.S. and Canada). Fax: 314-447-8029. E-mail: journalscustomerservice-usa@elsevier.com (for print support); journalsonlinesupport-usa@elsevier.com (for online support).**

Reprints. For copies of 100 or more, of articles in this publication, please contact the Commercial Reprints Department, Elsevier Inc., 360 Park Avenue South, New York, NY 10010-1710. Tel. 212-633-3874; Fax: 212-633-3820; E-mail: reprints@elsevier.com.

Physician Assistant Clinics is covered in *MEDLINE/PubMed (Index Medicus)* and *EMBASE/Excerpta Medica, Current Contents/Clinical Medicine, and ISI/BIOMED.*

Contributors

CONSULTING EDITOR

JAMES A. VAN RHEE, MS, PA-C, DFAAPA
Associate Professor, Program Director, Yale University, Yale Physician Associate Program, New Haven, Connecticut

EDITORS

KRISTYN S. LOWERY, MPA, PA-C
Department of Pediatric Cardiothoracic Surgery, Children's Hospital of Pittsburgh of UPMC, Pittsburgh, Pennsylvania

BRIAN R. WINGROVE, MHS, PA-C, DFAAPA
Children's Physician Group–Pulmonology, Scottish Rite, Children's Healthcare of Atlanta, Atlanta, Georgia

GENEVIEVE A.N. DELROSARIO, MHS, PA-C
Assistant Professor, Department of Physician Assistant Education, Saint Louis University; Physician Assistant, Cardinal Glennon Children's Medical Center, St. Louis, Missouri

AUTHORS

MEREDITH E. ALLEY, PA
Division of Urology, Children's Hospital of Philadelphia, Philadelphia, Pennsylvania

COURTNEY F. ANDRUS, MMS, PA-C, RD, LD
University Pediatric Associates, LLC, Washington University School of Medicine, St Louis, Missouri

JOHN ANSIAUX, MPH, CPSTI
Center for Childhood Injury Prevention, Texas Children's Hospital, Houston, Texas

CHRIS BARRY, PA-C, MMSc
Jeffers, Mann, & Artman Pediatrics, Raleigh, North Carolina

COURTNEY BISHOP, MPAS, PA-C
Physician Assistant, Department of Orthopaedics, Nationwide Children's Hospital; Secretary of Society for Physician Assistants in Pediatrics, Columbus, Ohio

KELLY J. BUTLER, MPAS, PA-C
Physician Assistant, Comprehensive Epilepsy Program, Children's Health, Children's Medical Center Dallas, Dallas, Texas

GENEVIEVE A.N. DELROSARIO, MHS, PA-C
Assistant Professor, Department of Physician Assistant Education, Saint Louis University; Physician Assistant, Cardinal Glennon Children's Medical Center, St. Louis, Missouri

ELIZABETH P. ELLIOTT, MS, PA-C
Physician Assistant Program, School of Allied Health, Baylor College of Medicine, Houston, Texas

AMY L. FLEMING, RD, MMS, PA-C
Physician Assistant, Vascular Surgery and Wound Care, Memorial Medical Group Vascular and Vein Surgery, Belleville, Illinois

HEATHER R. GILBREATH, MPAS, PA-C
Physician Assistant and Advanced Practice Manager, Children's Health; Clinical Instructor, UT Southwestern Medical Center, School of Health Professions, Dallas, Texas

AIMEE C. HARIRAMANI, MS, PA-C
Physician Assistant Program, School of Allied Health, Baylor College of Medicine, Houston, Texas

JENNIFER KRZMARZICK, PA-C
Emergency Services Inc., Columbus, Ohio

KRISTYN S. LOWERY, MPA, PA-C
Department of Pediatric Cardiothoracic Surgery, Children's Hospital of Pittsburgh of UPMC, Pittsburgh, Pennsylvania

ANNE WEISSLER, MMS, PA-C
Division of Dermatology, Department of Pediatrics, Cardinal Glennon Children's Hospital, Saint Louis University, St Louis, Missouri

BRIAN R. WINGROVE, MHS, PA-C, DFAAPA
Children's Physician Group–Pulmonology, Scottish Rite, Children's Healthcare of Atlanta, Atlanta, Georgia

Contents

Motor vehicle crashes (MVCs) are the leading cause of death among children aged 4 to 14 years, and the second leading cause of death among children aged 1 to 4 years. MVCs also result in 174,000 annual emergency room visits and 8000 hospitalizations of children up to age of 14 years. The American Academy of Pediatrics (AAP) and the National Highway Traffic Safety Administration have created evidence-based guidelines for child passenger safety (CPS), but compliance is still highly variable. CPS educational programs for future health care providers are greatly lacking, and many providers are unclear about the AAP guidelines.

The use of formula to supplement or replace breastfeeding is common in the United States. There are many formulations, brands, additives, and indications for the use of different formulas. Some are well founded in research, whereas the data are either conflicting or not well founded for others. This article provides a brief overview of the different types of formula that are commercially available and indications for their use.

Atrial septal defects are one of the most common types of congenital heart disease. Identified in infants to adults, there are varying degrees of symptoms with which patients may present. Types of atrial septal defects include ostium secundum, medicatie ostium primum, sinus venosus, and unroofed coronary sinus. Interventions include interventional cardiac catheterization, and cardiothoracic surgery; however, each therapy also includes potential complications.

Absence seizures were formerly called petit mal seizures, from the French, meaning little illness, implying a less severe seizure. However, these seizures can cause significant impairment, especially if untreated. Absence seizures often go unrecognized because they are brief and subtle. They are not characterized by convulsions and are often mistaken for daydreaming or inattention. The diagnosis is made by typical clinical history and electroencephalogram findings consistent with the condition. Several medications are effective in treating absence seizures. This article discusses diagnosis and management, beginning with some basic concepts and definitions before discussing the specifics of absence seizures and epilepsy.

Urinary tract infections (UTIs) are a fairly common occurrence in the pediatric population. Differentiating between cystitis and pyelonephritis is essential to determining type and duration of treatment as well as the appropriate workup. Appropriate radiologic imaging workup is discussed and is often based on level of UTI and age of the patient. Underlying anatomic abnormalities predisposing to a UTI are discussed and medical and surgical treatment options reviewed. Habits that can predispose to a UTI are reviewed and recommendations for optimal habits are made. Preventing UTIs is important to minimize exposure to antibiotics and ultimately important to protect renal health.

It may not kill you, but it can ruin your life. This describes the morbidity of uncontrolled atopic dermatitis, the most common chronic skin disease in children. Early identification and successful treatment may limit its extent. The American Academy of Dermatology updated clinical guidelines but admits gaps in research. Elidel and Protopic are approved for atopic dermatitis, along with topical and oral steroids. Limited options have made treatment frustrating. Clinical trials for topical and systemic therapies are in progress. Thought leaders have dubbed it a new dawn for atopic dermatitis. Information gathered may transform understanding and treatment.

Attention-deficit/hyperactivity disorder (ADHD) is the most common pediatric neurobehavioral disorder. Most individuals with ADHD have comorbid psychiatric illnesses, such as anxiety, depression, conduct disorder, or oppositional defiant disorder. Pediatric primary care providers are on the frontline for screening, evaluation, diagnosis, and management of childhood and adolescent ADHD. Stimulant medication has been considered first-line therapy for decades and continues to prove its efficacy among appropriately diagnosed patients. Nonstimulant medications and medical nutrition therapy have gained more recognition for either primary or supplemental management for ADHD. This article provides a clinical update on the screening, diagnostic guidelines, and management for pediatric primary care clinicians.

PHYSICIAN ASSISTANT CLINICS

THE CLINICS ARE AVAILABLE ONLINE!
Access your subscription at:
www.theclinics.com

Foreword

A Call for Preceptors

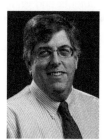

James A. Van Rhee, MS, PA-C, DFAAPA
Consulting Editor

All physician assistants need to read the editorial by Jennifer Krzmarzick regarding the need for clinical preceptors. My primary role now is program director for a physician assistant program and I hear from many programs of the shortage and need for additional clinical preceptors to train the physician assistants of the future.

Remember the preceptors you had while in school: the preceptor who sat down with you to explain EKGs or how to interpret an arterial blood gas; the preceptor who took time out of a busy day to explain the approach to a crying two-year-old who presented with ear pain; or the preceptor who helped you through the loss of your first patient. Before I went into academia, I precepted students for years in an inpatient internal medicine setting. I think it was working with these students that piqued my interest in education. Now is the time for you to be that receptor and have that impact on a PA student's career.

I know the reason people don't precept—the student slows me down, my practice doesn't allow it, or I won't meet my relative value unit (RVUs) for the month. All fair reasons, but whom better to teach the next generation of PAs than the current PAs in clinical practice? The 2013 AAPA Annual Report estimates there are over 93,000 physician assistants in clinical practice[1]; if each PA precepted at least one student per year, that would solve the preceptor crisis we are currently experiencing. Push your practice to take that one student; yes, it may slow you down, but the satisfaction you get from teaching and helping that one student will make up for any negative reasons you may have not to precept. I hear many practicing PAs say that the current training of PA students is not providing them with the skills they need for clinical practice; well here is your chance to step up and help. Be part of the solution.

This issue of *Physician Assistant Clinics* focuses on pediatrics, with a wide variety of topics. If you are practicing in pediatrics, primary care, or emergency medicine, there is something here for you.

Preventive medicine and safety are the focus of the article by Elliott, Hariramani and Ansiaux on child passenger safety, and Barry looks at the updates, changes, and complications in immunizations. Gilbreath provides an excellent review of common

Physician Assist Clin 1 (2016) xi–xii
http://dx.doi.org/10.1016/j.cpha.2016.08.002
2405-7991/16/© 2016 Published by Elsevier Inc.

neuromuscular disorders, such as muscular dystrophy, and Andrus gives us an update on attention-deficit/hyperactivity disorder for the primary care provider.

Nutrition is covered by Fleming and DelRosario as they help us make sense of infant feeding, with an article on the formula formulary. For those of you interested in cardiopulmonary disease, the articles by Lowery on atrial septal defects and Wingrove on pediatric asthma will be of interest. Bulter provides an excellent review of absence seizures, including etiologies and treatment.

I hope you enjoy the fourth issue of *Physician Assistant Clinics*. Our next issue will provide you with a review of the latest in endocrinology.

James A. Van Rhee, MS, PA-C, DFAAPA
Yale University
Yale Physician Assistant Program
100 Church Street South, Suite A250
New Haven, CT 06519, USA

E-mail address:
james.vanrhee@yale.edu

REFERENCE

1. American Academy of Physician Assistants. 2013 AAPA Annual Report. Available at: https://www.aapa.org/WorkArea/DownloadAsset.aspx?id=2902. Accessed August 3, 2016.

Preface

Widespread Role of Physician Assistants in Pediatrics

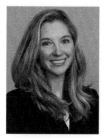 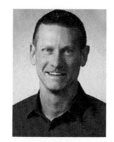 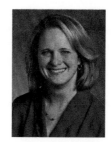

Kristyn S. Lowery, MPA, PA-C   Brian R. Wingrove, MHS, PA-C, DFAAPA   Genevieve A.N. DelRosario, MHS, PA-C

Editors

Since our inception, the purpose of physician assistants has been to increase access to quality medical care for everyone. The profession of Physician Assistant began to grow in the post-Vietnam era when a need for well-trained generalist medical providers was identified. In the late 1960s, Dr Henry Silver noted that many children were not receiving appropriate medical care. He went on to develop a 2- to 3-year program to train assistants for pediatricians, which he then called child health associates. With the concurrent growth of the physician assistant profession, these child health associates later evolved into physician assistants in pediatrics.

Today, there are over 3000 practicing physician assistants in pediatrics. Working in general pediatrics as well as almost every subspecialty, we provide care for all children from preterm infants through adolescents. We are proud to work together with pediatricians and other members of the health care team alongside families and children to improve children's health and well-being, preparing them for a healthy, wonderful life as they enter adulthood.

In this issue of *Physician Assistant Clinics*, our goal is to discuss a broad range of childhood health topics, including well-child care, neuromuscular disorders, asthma, congenital anomalies, and numerous others. Many pediatric physician assistants have come together in this issue to discuss the current evaluation, diagnostics, and management of various pediatric conditions. We would like to commend the Society of Physician Assistants in Pediatrics board and organization members for the research and time that were put into the development of each of these articles. We hope that you

Physician Assist Clin 1 (2016) xiii–xiv
http://dx.doi.org/10.1016/j.cpha.2016.08.001
2405-7991/16/   **physicianassistant.theclinics.com**

enjoy and learn from this issue as we work together to discover new ways that we can improve care for all children.

Kristyn S. Lowery, MPA, PA-C
Department of Pediatric Cardiothoracic Surgery
Children's Hospital of Pittsburgh of UPMC
4100 Penn Avenue
5th Floor, Faculty Pavilion
Pittsburgh, PA 15224, USA

Brian R. Wingrove, MHS, PA-C, DFAAPA
Children's Physician Group–
Pulmonology at Scottish Rite
Children's Healthcare of Atlanta
1100 Lake Hearn Drive, Suite 450
Atlanta, GA 30342, USA

Genevieve A.N. DelRosario, MHS, PA-C
Department of Physician Assistant Education
Saint Louis University
3437 Caroline Mall
St Louis, MO 63104-1111, USA

Cardinal Glennon Children's Medical Center
St. Louis, MO 63104-1095, USA

E-mail addresses:
Kristyn.lowery@chp.edu (K.S. Lowery)
brian.wingrove@choa.org (B.R. Wingrove)
gdelrosa@slu.edu (G.A.N. DelRosario)

Editorial: Calling All Preceptors

 CrossMark

Jennifer Krzmarzick, PA-C

Clinical rotations have always been a crucial component of any medical professional's education and their importance in the physician assistant (PA) curriculum is no exception. The Accreditation Review Commission on Education for the Physician Assistant (ARC-PA) has designed standards that PA programs must follow when creating their clinical rotation curriculum. One such standard is that students must have adequate exposure to patients of all ages, including infants, children, adults, and the elderly.[1] Although there is no specific standard that mandates schools to have a clinical rotation solely designated to pediatrics, PA programs generally incorporate a pediatric rotation into their curriculum because it is the easiest way to ensure that students achieve ARC-PA requirements.

Today there are 210 PA programs, with an additional 36 programs slated to open by July of 2018.[2] As the number of PA programs increases, so does the demand for clinical preceptors. The demand is, in fact, so high that it is often difficult for schools to find general pediatric rotations for all of their students. In some cases, schools are unable to place their students in a general pediatric rotation and are forced to substitute this experience for different types of rotations such as pediatric subspecialties or family practice rotations. Students can certainly benefit from these types of experiences, but it is no substitute for the knowledge and experience that can be gained from a general pediatric rotation.

This lack of preceptors not only can affect a student's education, but it could also affect the number of pediatric PAs in the workforce. According to the 2013 American Academy of Physician Assistants National Survey,[3] only 3.4% of the nearly 16,000 respondents work in pediatrics. Roughly two-thirds of these providers work in general pediatrics, and one-third work in subspecialties. This number is somewhat lower compared with other specialties within the PA profession. Having more PA students in pediatric hospitals and private practices can help expose other practitioners to the benefit of having a PA as part of a child's health care team.

With such an obvious need, there is an equally obvious answer: recruit more preceptors. The solution to this problem is much easier said than done. Preceptors rarely receive pay for their hard work and having a student is often time-consuming. However, a practitioner should also consider the benefits having a student. Precepting a student is a chance to give back to the PA community and to form relationships with future practitioners. It can also be a rewarding educational experience for themselves because students are taught the most up-to-date clinical practice knowledge and can share this with their providers. Preceptors can also be awarded up to 10 category 1 Continuing Medical Education hours per calendar year for volunteering to take

Emergency Services, Inc., 799 Thurber Dive West, Apartment #306, Columbus, OH 43215, USA
E-mail address: krzmarjm2@gmail.com

Physician Assist Clin 1 (2016) 523–524
http://dx.doi.org/10.1016/j.cpha.2016.06.003
2405-7991/16/$ – see front matter © 2016 Elsevier Inc. All rights reserved.
physicianassistant.theclinics.com

on a student.[4] There is even legislation currently being drafted by the American Academy of Physician Assistants and the Physician Assistant Education Association that would give preceptors an income tax exemption.[5]

As a recently graduated PA student, I thank all the pediatric PAs, physicians, and nurse practitioners who have generously given their time and talent to precept students. Your impact on a student's education and future career is immeasurable. For all pediatric practitioners, I urge you to consider taking on a student to help fill this great need within the PA community.

REFERENCES

1. Accreditation Review Commission on Education for Physician Assistants. Accreditation standards for physician assistant education. 4th edition. 2015.
2. Alesbury E. 11 New Programs Cleared to Enroll Students. 2016. Available at: http://paeaonline.org/11-new-programs-cleared-to-welcome-students/.
3. 2013 AAPA Annual Survey Report. American Academy of Physician Assistants; 2014.
4. American Academy of Physician Assistants. Category 1 CME for preceptors. 2016. Available at: https://www.aapa.org/twocolumnmain.aspx?id=1751.
5. Physician Assistant Education Association. Help preceptors catch a break – a tax break. Physician Assistant Education Association; 2016.

Child Passenger Safety

Elizabeth P. Elliott, MS, PA-C[a],*, Aimee C. Hariramani, MS, PA-C[a],
John Ansiaux, MPH, CPSTI[b]

KEYWORDS

- Car seat • Safety • Child restraint • Passenger • Vehicle

KEY POINTS

- Child passenger safety is an integral part of child safety, and anticipatory guidance regarding child passenger safety should be addressed at every well-child visit.
- Pediatric providers should familiarize themselves with the current American Academy of Pediatrics guidelines as well as safety topics pertaining to proper installation and use of car seats.
- Screening questions can be used by pediatric providers to identify potentially dangerous child passenger safety practices, and to target anticipatory guidance.
- Providers should refer all parents, but especially those failing installation screening questions, to a car seat technician.

INTRODUCTION

Motor vehicle crashes (MVCs) are the single leading cause of death in the US pediatric population among children aged 4 to 14 years, and the second leading cause of death among children aged 1 to 4 years, resulting in more than 1100 child deaths in 2013.[1] MVCs also accounted for nearly 8000 pediatric hospitalizations of children up to the age of 14 years, and 174,000 emergency department visits, all of which cost nearly $2.5 billion in medical and work loss costs.[2] For all of these reasons, with child safety chief among them, the American Academy of Pediatrics (AAP) and the National Highway Traffic Safety Administration (NHTSA) have consistently publicized policy recommendations and educational resources for the proper seating and restraint of children in motor vehicles through the age of 13 years. In order for children to be as safe as possible when riding in cars, parents must follow up-to-date AAP age-appropriate guidelines, must have child seats installed properly, and must use the seats properly every time a child is in the car (**Fig. 1**).

Disclosures: None.
[a] Physician Assistant Program, School of Allied Health, Baylor College of Medicine, One Baylor Plaza, Houston, Texas 77030, USA; [b] Center for Childhood Injury Prevention, Texas Children's Hospital, 1919 South Braeswood Boulevard, Suite 2228, Houston, TX, USA
* Corresponding author.
E-mail address: elliot@bcm.edu

Physician Assist Clin 1 (2016) 525–540
http://dx.doi.org/10.1016/j.cpha.2016.05.001
2405-7991/16/$ – see front matter © 2016 Elsevier Inc. All rights reserved.

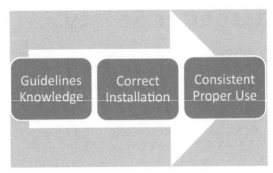

Fig. 1. Child passenger safety components.

Pediatric Motor Vehicle Crash Injuries

Serious injuries are strongly associated with nonrestraint or improper restraint of children in motor vehicles, including intra-abdominal injuries, as well as head, neck, and spinal cord injuries. Abdominal wall bruising or lap-belt ecchymosis, is a common finding associated with improper restraint use, and can indicate a likelihood of abdominal injuries, vertebral fractures, and spinal cord injury (**Fig. 2**).[3]

In a 3-year pediatric trauma study, 46 patients were found to have abdominal wall ecchymosis, and nearly half of them had to undergo exploratory surgery. Of those 46 children, only 1 was restrained using a 5-point harness per the AAP age-specific guidelines. All others were wearing a seat belt only.[4]

Child Passenger Safety Guidelines

Before the 1970s, children of all ages rode in motor vehicles either completely unrestrained or restrained with the car seat belts, often a single lap belt only, and child MVC morbidities and mortalities were high. Even now, unrestrained children are at the highest risk of morbidity and mortality, having greater than 3 times the risk of injury compared with properly restrained children.[5]

The first child safety seats were created and sold in the United States in the 1970s, and the AAP first began issuing recommendations for parent education and legislation

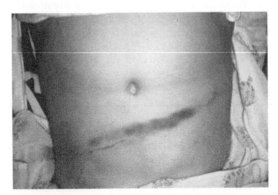

Fig. 2. Lap belt ecchymosis. (*Reprinted from* Muñiz A. Evaluation and management of pediatric abdominal trauma. Pediatr Emerg Med Pract 2008;5(3); with permission from EB Medicine; and *Courtesy of* Dr Antonio Muñiz.)

for child passenger safety (CPS) in 1981.[6] Once the use of child restraints gained momentum, the incidence of pediatric injury and death attributed to MVCs began to decline. The most recent AAP Guidelines for Child Passenger Safety were issued in 2011, specifying evidence-based criteria for the proper restraint of children from birth to age 13 years.[7]

The guidelines may be summarized as follows:

- Until a minimum age of 2 years, children should be restrained in a rear-facing car seat in the back seat.
- After age 2 years, or after a child has outgrown rear-facing height and weight limits, the child should be restrained in a forward-facing car seat in the back seat until a minimum age of 4 years.
- After age 4 years, or after a child has outgrown forward-facing height and weight limits, the child should be restrained in the back seat in a booster seat that correctly positions the car's safety belt system on the child's body.
- Once children reach 145 cm (57″) tall (typically between the ages of 8 and 12 years), they can safely discontinue use of the booster seat and be restrained with the rear lap and shoulder seat belts of a car until a minimum age of 13 years.
- After the age of 13 years, children may safely ride in the front seat of a vehicle while wearing a lap and shoulder seat belt (**Fig. 3**).

Per the AAP Committee on Injury, Violence, and Poison Prevention, age-appropriate guidelines are designed to reduce injury by reducing risk of ejection, distributing energy of the crash over bony anatomy, and limiting contact of the passenger with interior vehicle structures.[7] In addition, the guidelines take into account age-specific anatomic features. For example, with children less than 2 years of age, the head is proportionally larger than the neck, cervical ligaments are lax, and vertebrae are not completely ossified. This anatomy puts children at this age at increased risk for head and cervical spinal cord injury, especially when facing forward. In contrast, a rear-facing seat can distribute crash forces away from the head and neck.[7] Henary and colleagues[8] showed that rear-facing car seats were 5 times more effective than forward-facing car seats in preventing serious injury or death between the ages of 1 and 2 years. It has also been shown that, in general, rear-facing car seats reduce the incidence of injury, the risk of severe injury, and the weight load on the neck in a motor vehicle crash (**Fig. 4**).

When guidelines are followed correctly, estimates have shown reduced risk of injury by as much as 82%,[9,10] and reduced risk of death by up to 45% compared with seat belts alone.[11,12] Within the last year, 3 states (California, Oklahoma, and New Jersey) have used the AAP and NHTSA guidelines in passing legislation requiring that children be rear facing until 2 years of age. Other states, such as Oregon and Texas, are working on similar legislation. The evidence serving as the foundation for this legislation is not privy just to legislators but needs to be disseminated to all family seen during well-child examinations.

Lack of Compliance with Child Passenger Safety Policies

Although AAP age-specific guidelines are intended to advise parents and families, there is no consistent way of disseminating this information to the public at large, often leaving parents with information that is no longer up to date. A survey of parents who used convertible car seats was conducted by a car seat manufacturer, Chicco. It showed that 58% of parents did not know the minimum age at which a car seat should be changed to forward facing.[13] In another study, by O'Neil and colleagues[14] in 2012,

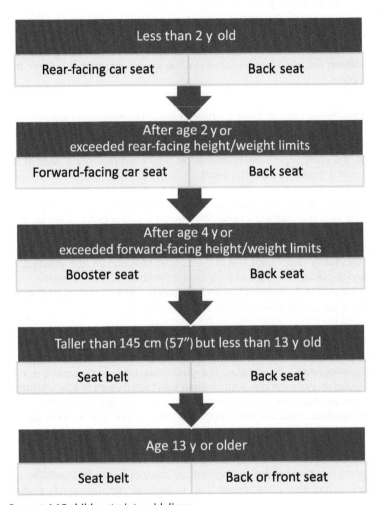

Fig. 3. Current AAP child restraint guidelines.

only 62% of parents of children less than 2 years of age knew that the rear-facing position was safer. In contrast, guideline-appropriate use of car seats and booster seats has been correlated with parental knowledge about age, height, and weight recommendations.[15] Education is therefore essential in order for parents to follow guidelines; however, it is not sufficient.

In the Chicco study, approximately one-third of parents reported that they did not follow manufacturer safety guidelines regarding when to turn car seats to forward facing, and 49% of parents made the decision to turn their children based on comfort rather than safety.[13] Another study showed that as few as 1 in 5 children between the ages of 1 and 2 years were correctly observed to be in the rear-facing position, increasing their chances of serious injuries.[14] According to Agran and colleagues,[16] both lack of knowledge and perception of low risk of injury and death have been barriers to using child safety seats as recommended. Of most concern is that studies estimate that approximately 20% of parents are not using child restraint at all.[17,18]

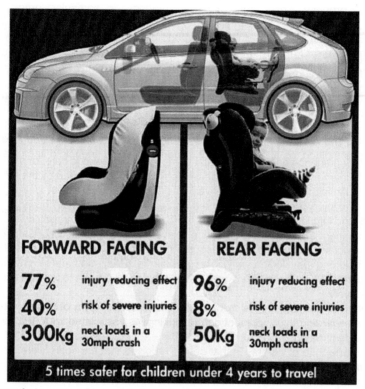

FORWARD FACING

77%	injury reducing effect
40%	risk of severe injuries
300Kg	neck loads in a 30mph crash

REAR FACING

96%	injury reducing effect
8%	risk of severe injuries
50Kg	neck loads in a 30mph crash

5 times safer for children under 4 years to travel

Fig. 4. Rear-facing versus forward-facing injury risk. (*Courtesy of* Securatot Ltd, Brinkworth, UK; with permission.)

In a large observational study of 21,476 children, decreased use of child safety seats and increased incidence of nonrestraint were linearly associated with increasing child age.[19] Less than 30% of children 8 to 12 years old shorter than 145 cm (57″) tall were restrained in a booster seat as prescribed by the guidelines, putting the other 70% at significantly increased risk for injury or death.[19]

Improper Installation and Use of Car Seats

Even if parents are educated about guidelines and are eager to comply with them, the tedious car seat installation process can be a barrier to proper use of a child safety seat. The Chicco study found that 19% of parents found installation of their car seat difficult and 40% found it overwhelming.[13] However, only 15% of parents sought professional assistance with installation.[13] Another study showed that up to 80% of parents used child safety seats incorrectly.[17] These data suggest that parents require education regarding proper car seat installation, in addition to safety guidelines.

Once the child safety seat is installed properly, the child must also be harnessed into the seat properly. Per the AAP, shoulder harness straps should insert at or below shoulder level in rear-facing seats, and at or above shoulder level in forward-facing seats. Chest clips should be located at the level of the axillae. In addition, all harnesses should be completely flat and without slack.[20]

The proper installation and use of child safety seats is complicated, and parents require guidance about how to keep their children safe. Certified car seat technicians are able to help with such detailed instruction. However, pediatric providers should be willing and able to provide basic information about AAP guidelines and standards for proper installation and use, as well as resources for additional help, because providers have a unique and powerful role in being able to help prevent childhood injury.[20–22] In addition, pediatric providers should be able to use their knowledge and resources regarding CPS to adequately screen patients and families who might be at risk for improper installation and/or use of their car seats in motor vehicles.

The Role of the Pediatric Provider in Increasing Rates of Compliance and Proper Use

Anticipatory guidance has been a pivotal component of pediatric care for many years and is a fundamental component of the well-child check, as detailed by the Affordable Care Act. Anticipatory guidance serves to educate families about developmental changes and injury prevention associated with particular ages. Given the large number of deaths and injuries attributed to MVCs, CPS education is encouraged by the AAP to be a component of anticipatory guidance at every well-child check. Parents routinely cite pediatricians as being primary resources for CPS information.[14,23] Pediatric providers, including physicians, physician assistants (PAs), and nurse practitioners, should therefore be trained to provide this anticipatory guidance to families accurately and effectively.

Morrongiello and colleagues[23] studied the difference in provider and parent perspectives regarding injury prevention counseling. Physicians were found to significantly overestimated the amount of time they spent addressing issues of safety. Less than one-third of parents in that cohort reported that car seats were discussed with them by their children's physician. Parents were also reluctant to bring up topics of safety, with 64% stating that they had rarely or never asked such questions. This study shows that, if providers are not offering, many parents are not asking. However, 82% of parents indicated that, if their child's physician spent more time on issues of safety, they would be likely to follow the advice of the physician and make changes accordingly.[23]

Multiple studies have documented variable knowledge and attitudes of pediatricians regarding CPS.[24,25] Furthermore, provision of information to parents regarding CPS tends to be more standard with infants and toddlers and decreases in frequency for school-aged children, although AAP guidelines affect children until 13 years of age.[24] According to O'Neil and colleagues,[14] only half of parents recalled having had a conversation with their child's health care provider about child passenger safety. Those who had were more likely to follow the recommendation of keeping their child rear facing until a minimum age of 2 years. For older children, booster seat counseling was acknowledged by pediatricians to be an important strategy for injury prevention. However, 39% of providers reported that they did not counsel parents about booster seats unless it was the explicit reason for the office visit, and only 52% have counseled at least half of their families about booster seats.[14]

Provider Lack of Knowledge Regarding Child Passenger Safety

Although many barriers and competing priorities contribute to undersharing of CPS information, one that can be combated in the professional training period is lack of knowledge. Although the AAP sees CPS as a critical topic of anticipatory guidance, CPS curriculum has rarely been part of medical education for medical students, PA students, or residents.[23,26] According to one study at the Children's National Medical Center, less than one-fourth of pediatric residents had ever heard a lecture about CPS, and less than a third were comfortable talking about CPS with families.[26] In another study, 63% of physicians surveyed stated that medical school had not prepared them for injury prevention counseling.[23]

One particularly relevant study by Zonfrillo and colleagues[24] evaluated pediatrician knowledge of CPS and gathered information regarding dissemination of CPS information at well-child visits. In this study with 533 participants, only half of respondents were able to answer all questions accurately. These high-knowledge respondents were more likely to discuss CPS with parents in person (rather than distributing printed resources), address the topic with more frequency, have higher levels of confidence about the topic, and cite fewer barriers to delivery compared with the control.

Emergency medicine providers are also poised to provide accurate CPS recommendations to families in the emergency department (ED) after an MVC. Two recent studies showed that, even though ED physicians see value in providing CPS information to families, they cite lack of knowledge as the primary barrier to doing so, resulting in irregular and infrequent dissemination of the information.[27,28] One study showed low ED provider CPS pretest knowledge, which significantly improved after a brief CPS educational intervention.[29] These studies suggest that ED providers are interested and willing to provide CPS information to families but require more education in order to be able to do so.

The Need for Child Passenger Safety Education for Providers

According to previous studies, parents are likely to turn to their pediatric providers first with questions about child passenger safety[14] and how to prevent injuries in childhood.[23] This finding shows the urgent need for CPS education during medical education programs. Furthermore, because guidelines are updated frequently, the need continues to be present in continuing medical education (CME) programs for pediatric providers in clinical practice.

With provisions in the Affordable Care Act calling for advanced practice providers to help increase access to primary and preventive care, it is essential that PAs also be educated in the fundamentals of CPS so they may guide families and answer pertinent questions on the topics of child safety and injury prevention. Whether working in the fields of pediatrics, community medicine, or emergency medicine, PAs play an essential role in educating parents so that accidental deaths and injuries may be prevented.

CLINICAL PRACTICE
The Pediatric Visit

As stated previously, anticipatory guidance is an integral part of pediatric patient care, during both the acute and well-child visits. Pediatric providers in many settings are in a position to provide vital information to families regarding CPS. However, providers often lack knowledge or skill in asking the appropriate questions to determine whether or not the child is properly restrained in a motor vehicle. *Bright Futures* from the AAP is a helpful resource that providers can use as a starting point. Information regarding CPS is listed under each well-child visit, divided by age. Although not comprehensive, this resource gives questions that can help identify basic areas of risk with regard to CPS, along with anticipatory guidance statements that can help guide parent education.[30] Two additional resources are the AAP's "Car Seat Checkup" and "Car Safety Seats: Information for Families," which can be found on the AAP Web site (www.healthychildren.org).[20,21] **Fig. 5** shows the AAP's best-practice recommendations for CPS. The AAP has also created a mobile device

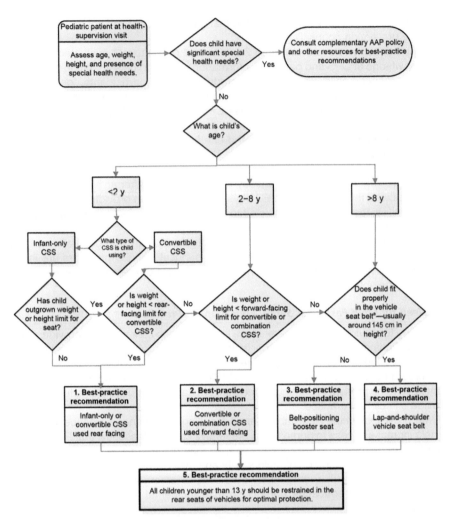

Fig. 5. AAP best-practice recommendations for child passenger safety. CSS, child safety seat. (*Data from* American Academy of Pediatrics policy statement – child passenger safety. Available at: http://pediatrics.aappublications.org/content/pediatrics/early/2011/03/21/peds.2011-0213.full.pdf. Accessed February 25, 2016.)

app called CarSeatCheck. The app includes a seat checker to help select the correct seat for a specific child, a product guide with height and weight limits, a section on installation help, and safety information that includes assistance with finding a technician.[31]

An Orientation to Child Safety Seats and Current American Academy of Pediatrics Guidelines

The current child safety seat market has many options for parents. It is important that pediatric providers be familiar with the general types of car seats available to parents so that they can address issues specific to that seat. **Fig. 6** shows an example of an infant carrier. These seats generally have a base that is installed securely in the

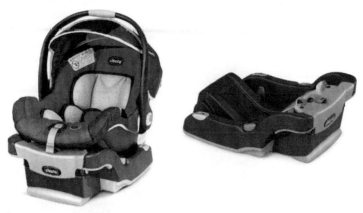

Fig. 6. Infant carrier seat (Chicco USA, Lancaster PA).

vehicle. The infant is properly secured in the seat and the seat locks into the base for transport in the motor vehicle. These seats may be used from birth until the child outgrows the height and weight limits provided by the manufacturer for the specific seat.

Fig. 7 shows an example of a convertible car seat. These seats may be used in the rear-facing or forward-facing position. The manufacturer provides rear-facing and forward-facing height and weight limits for these seats. This seat should be used in a rear-facing position until at least 2 years of age, and preferably longer if the child has not outgrown the rear-facing weight or height limits for the seat.

After the minimum age of 4 years, and after the child has outgrown the limits of the convertible car seat, the child is ready for a combination seat or booster seat. In **Fig. 8**, a combination seat with a 5-point harness is shown. A combination seat converts from a forward-facing seat with a harness to a booster after the child

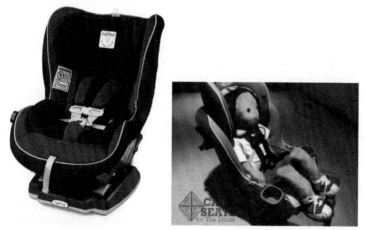

Fig. 7. Convertible car seat with proper placement of child in seat. (*Courtesy of* Car Seats for the Littles, Inc.; with permission)

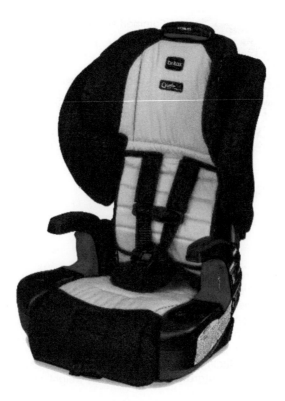

Fig. 8. Combination seat with 5-point harness. (*Courtesy of* Britax, Fort Mill, SC; with permission.)

exceeds the harness' maximum height or weight. Again, choosing a combination seat with a 5-point harness provides more protection in the case of a collision, because the harness distributes the force of the crash more evenly across the child's body.

Fig. 9 shows an example of a booster seat. It may have a back or be backless. These seats are also an option when the child has outgrown a rear-facing or forward-facing seat. However, they do not have the 5-point harness. In these seats, the child needs to be restrained by the vehicle's seat belt. Note that most booster seats have a minimum height, weight, or age requirement. Many booster seats require that the child be at least 4 years of age to use a booster seat. The vehicle seat belt must be properly aligned on the child's body in order for this type of booster seat to be safe. The shoulder belt should cross the middle of the clavicle without touching the neck. In addition, the lap belt should fit across the child's hips, without crossing the abdomen.

Beyond the Guidelines

Although the AAP guidelines (see **Fig. 3**) provide general guidance about CPS and suggested ages for the use of different child safety seats, they do not give information for health care providers regarding screening for proper car seat safety use and installation. With about 80% of car safety seats being used

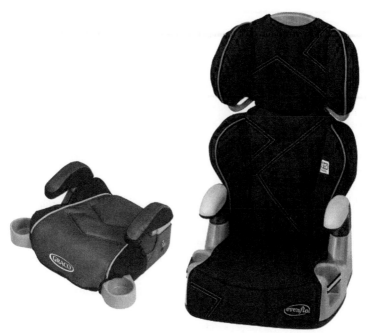

Fig. 9. Booster seat. (*Courtesy of* Evenflo Company, Inc, Miamisburg, Ohio and Graco Children's Products Inc, High Point, NC.)

incorrectly,[17] it is imperative that pediatric providers know more than just the AAP guidelines. Pediatric providers need to be able to assess the family's use of child safety seats and knowledge of CPS to determine whether the family requires referral to a car seat technician for education regarding proper installation and use of the seat (visit www.seatcheck.org for more information). Parents often do not realize that they are using and/or installing the seats incorrectly, so it is imperative that pediatric providers play a role in this integral aspect of child safety.

Child Passenger Safety Screening

In addition to the guidance provided by *Bright Futures* and AAP printable materials, **Box 1** shows useful screening questions to be used to assess proper installation and use of car safety seats along with parent and patient knowledge regarding CPS.

When screening a parent or patient for proper implementation of CPS guidelines, note that not all of the questions in **Box 1** apply at every visit. Providers should be aware of the AAP and NHTSA guidelines for the age/size of the child and be able to apply these questions to the specific situation, with the goal of keeping each child in the safest car seat for that child's weight and height for as long as possible. For example, just because a child reaches 2 years of age does not mean that a forward-facing car seat is the safest option. The child may still be more appropriately and safely restrained in a rear-facing seat if the child has not outgrown the height and weight limits. Also, just because a child is tall enough to use a booster seat does not mean that child should discontinue use of a 5-point harness. **Box 2** lists the proper

---

Box 1
Screening questions for parents and patients regarding proper car seat knowledge, installation, and use

Basic knowledge and driving habits

Are all passengers always restrained in the car while the vehicle is moving?

How many car safety seats and booster seats are installed in your vehicle?

Is any driver ever under the influence of alcohol or drugs while your child is a passenger in the vehicle?

Are there any other distractions in the car for drivers (eg, mobile devices, child mirrors, navigation screens, loud music)?

Guidelines knowledge

Do you know when to convert from an infant carrier to a rear-facing convertible car seat?

Do you know when to convert from a rear-facing to a forward-facing car seat?

Do you know when to convert from a forward-facing car seat to a booster seat?

Do you know when it will be safe for your child to be restrained by the seat belt only (no booster seat)?

Do you know when it will be safe for your child to ride in the front seat of a vehicle?

Installation

What type of seat do you use for your child (ie, infant carrier, convertible seat, booster seat)?

Where is the child safety seat installed in the car (eg, front seat, back seat, middle seat)?

Is the child safety seat rear facing or forward facing?

Do you know the height and weight limits of your current car seat?

Does your booster seat have a 5-point harness?

Did you use a seat belt or LATCH (lower anchors and tethers for children) system to install your car seat?

Has your seat installation been inspected by a car seat technician?

How much does the base of the seat move when forcibly moving the seat side to side (using a lateral force of 7 kg [15 lb])?

Is the seat wedged against any other child safety seat, or any other part of the vehicle?

Use

When the child is restrained in the car seat, what is the child wearing?

Do you put blankets under the buckles when the baby is cold?

Where is the chest clip secured on the child's body?

How loose are the straps on the car seat when the child is restrained in the seat?

Are there any products installed on your car seat (eg, covers, toys, mirrors, neck supports)?

---

guidance with regard to child safety in the context of the questions in **Box 1**. If an answer to a screening question is not among the answers given later, the provider needs to educate parents on relevant CPS practices. If the issue involves improper installation of the car safety seat, the family should be referred to a car seat technician through www.seatcheck.org.

Box 2

Appropriate answers to screening questions for CPS

Basic knowledge and driving habits

- Are all passengers always restrained in the car while the vehicle is moving?
  - ○ All passengers should be properly restrained in the motor vehicle. This behavior models the expectation as the child grows.
- How many car safety seats and booster seats are installed in your vehicle?
  - ○ Depending on the type of vehicle the family uses, this number varies. No two seats should be touching to the point that one is wedged under another.
- Is any driver under the influence of alcohol or drugs while your child is a passenger in the vehicle?
  - ○ No influence of alcohol or drugs should be permitted by any driver in any vehicle in which your child is a passenger.
- Are there any other distractions in the car for drivers?
  - ○ Mobile devices, extra mirrors, loud music, navigation screens, and aftermarket child entertainment and comfort devices can all be distractions to drivers of children.

Guidelines knowledge

- Do you know when to convert from an infant carrier to a rear-facing convertible car seat?
  - ○ If a child exceeds the height or weight maximum or is 1 year old, the child should transition from an infant carrier into a convertible seat. Parents are able to transition most children into convertible seats long before a turning seat, because most convertible car seats accommodate children starting at 2.3 kg (5 lb).
- Do you know when to convert from a rear-facing to a forward-facing car seat?
  - ○ When the toddler outgrows the weight or height limits of a rear-facing car seat (at least 2 years of age). However, the longer a child can stay rear facing, the safer that child will be while traveling in a motor vehicle.
- Do you know when to convert from a forward-facing car seat to a booster seat?
  - ○ Children can transition from a forward-facing car seat to a booster seat once they exceed the height or weight limit of a forward-facing car seat (at least 4 years of age). In addition, if a child exceeds the height or weight of the current seat, but is not mature enough to handle a booster seat, it may be appropriate to look for a forward-facing seat with a higher height and weight maximum.
- Do you know when it will be safe for your child to be restrained by the seat belt only (ie, no booster seat)?
  - ○ The car seat belt begins to fit children best when they are at least 145 cm (57 inches) tall. The shoulder portion of the seat belt should sit across midclavicle and the lap portion rests across the hips.
- Do you know when it will be safe for your child to ride in the front seat of a vehicle?
  - ○ When the child is 13 years old.

Installation

- What type of seat do you use for your child (ie, infant carrier, convertible seat, booster seat)?
  - ○ Depending on the age/weight/height of the child and the weight and height limits of the seat, the correct answer to this question varies.
- Where is the child safety seat installed in the car (eg, front seat, back seat, middle seat)?
  - ○ The safety seat should always be installed in the rear seat of the vehicle, preferably in the middle seat.
- Is the child safety seat rear facing or forward facing?
  - ○ Depending on the age/weight/height of the child and the weight and height limits of the seat, the correct answer to this question varies. However, all children less than 2 years of age should be rear facing.

- Do you know the height and weight limits of your current car seat?
  - This answer varies by style of seat and manufacturer. The information can be found in the original car seat manual or in an online manual.
- Does your booster seat have a 5-point harness?
  - Children should be restrained with a 5-point harness as long as possible, until the child outgrows the height and weight limits of the harness as suggested by the manufacturer. A 5-point harness distributes the weight in an accident over more surface area, reducing injury.
- Do you use a seat belt or LATCH system to install your car seat?
  - Car safety seats should be properly installed using a seat belt or LATCH system, but not both. All LATCH systems also have weight limits, which must be followed for the seat to be safely installed. This information can be found in the original car seat manual, the vehicle manual, or an online manual.
- Has your seat installation been inspected by a car seat technician?
  - More than 80% of seats are improperly installed by parents. Inspection by a car seat technician can help ensure proper installation.
- How much does the base of the seat move when forcibly moving the seat side to side (lateral force of 7 kg [15 lb])?
  - The base of the car seat should not move more than 2.5 cm (1 inch) laterally when pulled with 7 kg (15 lb) of force in a lateral direction.
- Is the seat wedged against any other child safety seat, or any other part of the vehicle?
  - The car seat should not be wedged against a door, other car safety seat, or backs of the other seats in the vehicle.

Use

- When the child is restrained in the car seat, what is the child wearing?
  - The child should be wearing a thin single layer of clothes. Bulky clothing should never be worn under the buckles of a car safety seat.
- Do you put blankets under the buckles when the baby is cold?
  - Blankets should be placed over the top of the buckles if the baby is cold.
- Where is the chest clip secured on the child's body?
  - The chest clip should be secured at the level of the axilla (see **Fig. 7**).
- How loose are the straps on the car seat when the child is restrained in the seat?
  - The parent should not be able to pinch any slack at the level of the shoulder when the child is properly restrained in a child safety seat (see **Fig. 7**).
- Are there any products installed on your car seat (ie, covers, toys, mirrors, neck supports)?
  - There are no nonregulated products that are approved for installation on any car seats (eg, car seat covers, mirrors, toys). These products all void the car seat warranty and can affect the safety of the seat. Aftermarket devices can also become projectiles, injuring children in an MVC.

SUMMARY

Although great progress have been made since the advent of child safety seats, there is still significant morbidity and mortality associated with MVCs in the pediatric patient population. Despite efforts on the part of the AAP and NHTSA to publish guidelines, most car safety seats are still improperly installed and misused, putting those children at risk for injury or death. This situation makes CPS essential and integral to well-child care. As such, it should be discussed at every well-child visit, especially given that parents consistently choose their providers as the preferred sources of information on child safety. Many providers now think that they are ill-prepared to address CPS issues with patients and families. Integration of this material into medical education and CME is vital to increasing CPS knowledge among providers. In addition, a brief review of AAP guidelines, the use of AAP resources such as *Bright Futures*, and the implementation of some routine screening questions can make all providers well-equipped to address this critical safety topic. When pediatric providers make CPS a priority, they take the first step toward building a future in which pediatric MVC morbidity and mortality statistics continue to decline, and children become adequately protected against unnecessary childhood injuries and loss of life.

REFERENCES

1. Centers for Disease Control and Prevention. Ten leading causes of injury deaths by age group highlighting unintentional injury deaths, United States. Available at: http://www.cdc.gov/injury/images/lc-charts/leading_causes_of_injury_deaths_highlighting_unintentional_injury_deaths_2013-a.gif. Accessed July 8, 2015.

2. CDC, Injury prevention & control: data & statistics. Web-based Injury Statistics Query and Reporting System (WISQARS TM), cost of injury reports, 2013. Accessed July 13, 2015.

3. Achildi O, Betz RR, Grewal H. Lapbelt injuries and the seatbelt syndrome in pediatric spinal cord injury. J Spinal Cord Med 2007;30:S21–4.

4. Campbell DJ, Sprouse LR, Smith LA, et al. Injuries in pediatric patients with seatbelt contusions. Am Surg 2003;69(12):1095–9.

5. Durbin DR, Chen I, Smith R, et al. Effects of seating position and appropriate restraint use on the risk of injury to children in motor vehicle crashes. Pediatrics 2005;155(3):e305–9.

6. Stewart DD, editor. More than forty years of progress for child passenger protection: a chronicle of child passenger safety advances in the USA, 1965-2009. 2009. p. 206. Document 364-5696. Available at: www.saferidenews.com. Accessed July 16, 2015.

7. Durbin DR, Committee on Injury, Violence, and Poison Prevention. Child passenger safety. Pediatrics 2011;127:e1050–66.

8. Henary B, Sherwood C, Crandall J, et al. Car safety seats for children: rear facing for best protection. Inj Prev 2007;13:398–402.

9. Arbogast KB, Durbin DR, Cornejo RA, et al. An evaluation of the effectiveness of forward facing child restraint systems. Accid Anal Prev 2004;36(4):585–9.

10. Zaloshnja E, Miller TR, Hendrie D. Effectiveness of child safety seats vs safety belts for children aged 2 to 3 years. Arch Pediatr Adolesc Med 2007;161(1):65–8.

11. Arbogast KB, Jermakian JS, Kallan MJ, et al. Effectiveness of belt positioning booster seats: an updated assessment. Pediatrics 2009;124:1281–6.

12. Elliott RM, Kallan MJ, Durbin DR, et al. Effectiveness of child safety seats vs seat belts in reducing risk for death in children in passenger vehicle crashes. Arch Pediatr Adolesc Med 2006;160(6):617–21.

13. Chicco USA. New national survey reveals majority of parents do not follow car seat safety guidelines. Available at: http://www.prnewswire.com/news-releases/new-national-survey-reveals-majority-of-parents-do-not-follow-car-seat-safety-guidelines-224406371.html. Accessed July 16, 2015.

14. O'Neil J, Slaven JE, Talty J, et al. Are parents following the recommendations of keeping children younger than 2 years rear facing during motor vehicle travel? Inj Prev 2014;20:226–31.

15. Bilston LE, Finch C, Hatfield J, et al. Age-specific parental knowledge of restraint transitions influences appropriateness of child occupant restraint use. Inj Prev 2008;14:159–63.

16. Agran PF, Anderson CL, Winn DG. Violators of a child passenger safety law. Pediatrics 2004;114(1):109–15.

17. Biagioli F. Proper use of child safety seats. Am Fam Physician 2002;65(10): 2085–90.

18. National Highway Safety Administration. The National Occupant Protection Use Survey. 2013.

19. Macy ML, Freed GL. Child passenger safety practices in the US: disparities in light of updated recommendations. Am J Prev Med 2012;43(3):272–81.

20. American Academy of Pediatrics. Car safety seats: information for families. 2016. Available at: https://www.healthychildren.org/English/safety-prevention/on-the-go/Pages/Car-Safety-Seats-Information-for-Families.aspx. Accessed February 27, 2016.

21. American Academy of Pediatrics. Car seat checkup. 2016. Available at: https://www.healthychildren.org/English/safety-prevention/on-the-go/Pages/Car-Safety-Seat-Checkup.aspx. Accessed February 27, 2016.

22. Micik S, Alpert J. The pediatrician as advocate. Pediatr Clin North Am 1985;31: 243–9.

23. Morrongiello BA, Hillier L, Bass M. 'What I said' versus 'what you heard': a comparison of physicians' and parents' reporting of anticipatory guidance on child safety issues. Inj Prev 1995;1:223–7.

24. Zonfrillo MF, Sauber-Schatz EK, Hoffman BD, et al. Pediatricians' self-reported knowledge, attitudes and practices about child passenger safety. J Pediatr 2014;165:1040–5.

25. Yingling F, Stombaught HA, Jeffrey J, et al. Pediatricians' knowledge, perceptions, and behaviors regarding car booster seats. J Community Health 2011; 36:166–73.

26. Tender JAF, Taft CH, Frey C, et al. Pediatric residents buckle up: a child safety seat training program for pediatric residents. Ambul Pediatr 2001;1:333–7.

27. Zonfrillo MR, Nelson KA, Durbin DR. Emergency physicians' knowledge and provision of child passenger safety information. Acad Emerg Med 2011;18:145–51.

28. Macy ML, Clark SJ, Sasson C, et al. Emergency physician perspectives on child passenger safety: a national survey of attitudes and practices. Acad Pediatr 2012;12:131–7.

29. Ekundayo OJ, Jones G, Brown A, et al. A brief educational intervention to improve healthcare providers' awareness of child passenger safety. Int J Pediatr 2013; 2013:821693.

30. Hagan JF, Shaw JS, Duncan PM, editors. Bright futures: guidelines for health supervision of infants, children, and adolescents. 3rd edition. Elk Grove Village (IL): American Academy of Pediatrics; 2008.

31. American Academy of Pediatrics. CarSeatCheck App, version 1.2. Created in 2013. 2014. Accessed February 27, 2016.

Formula Formulary
Making Sense of Infant Feeding

Amy L. Fleming, RD, MMS, PA-C[a],*, Genevieve A.N. DelRosario, MHS, PA-C[b,c]

KEYWORDS

- Formula nutrients • Infant formula • Soy formula
- Long-chain polyunsaturated fatty acids • Probiotics • Cow's milk allergy
- Modified protein formula

KEY POINTS

- When breastfeeding is not an option, healthy term infants should be placed on a standard formula unless there is a specific medical indication.
- Caregivers and providers should remain skeptical of claims made by formula companies, because many marketing claims have little supporting evidence.
- Specialized formulas are available for a variety of different medical indications.
- Many formulas now contain additives, such as long-chain polyunsaturated fatty acids, prebiotics, probiotics, and synbiotics. Although there is no known harm from these products, most research fails to find significant benefit. Additional investigation is warranted.

INTRODUCTION

The use of formula to supplement or replace breastfeeding is commonplace in the United States due to both medical reasons and personal preferences. However, the choice of formula may be confusing for patients and providers alike. There are many formulations, brands, additives, and indications for the use of different formulas. Parents may also confuse normal infant behavior such as spitting up and straining for a formula intolerance. In this article, the authors provide a brief overview of the different types of formula that are commercially available and indications for their use.

BREAST MILK AND ADVANTAGES OF BREASTFEEDING

A full discussion of infant formula is incomplete without the understanding that breastfeeding is the gold standard for infant feeding. The American Academy of Pediatrics (AAP) recommends "exclusive breastfeeding for about six months, followed by

The authors have nothing to disclose.
[a] Vascular Surgery and Wound Care, Memorial Medical Group Vascular and Vein Surgery, 4600 Memorial Drive, Suite 120, Bldg B, Belleville, IL 62226, USA; [b] Department of Physician Assistant Education, Saint Louis University, 3437 Caroline Mall, St. Louis, MO 63104-1111, USA; [c] Cardinal Glennon Children's Medical Center, St. Louis, MO 63104-1095, USA
* Corresponding author.
E-mail address: amy242526@gmail.com

Physician Assist Clin 1 (2016) 541–552
http://dx.doi.org/10.1016/j.cpha.2016.05.003
2405-7991/16/$ – see front matter © 2016 Elsevier Inc. All rights reserved.

continued breastfeeding as complementary foods are introduced, with continuation of breastfeeding for one year or longer as mutually desired by mother and infant."[1] The World Health Organization's position is similar, recommending 6 months of exclusive breastfeeding followed by breast milk in combination with complementary foods through 23 months of life.[2]

There are many documented advantages of breastfeeding. Infants who are breastfed experience fewer episodes of otitis media and lower rates of respiratory tract infections.[1] Research has suggested that infants who are breastfed have lower rates of sudden infant death; less allergic disease; decreased risk of developing obesity, type 1 and 2 diabetes; as well as lower risk for developing cardiovascular disease later in life.[1,3] Breastfeeding for greater than 3 months has been shown to result in improved intelligence and neurodevelopmental outcomes, particularly in high-risk populations such as infants born prematurely.[1]

Despite these guidelines, the use of infant formula is commonplace in the United States. In 2012, almost 20% of infants received formula in the first days of life, with greater than a third of infants receiving supplementation before first 6 months. By 1 year of age, just over 20% of infants received any breast milk, suggesting formula use may continue to increase in the second 6 months of life.[4] Thus, it is critical that the pediatric clinician has an appropriate understanding of its use.

OVERVIEW: PREPARATIONS AND NUTRIENTS

Commercially prepared infant formulas are designed to mimic the nutritional content and bioavailability of breast milk and should be offered in cases where breastfeeding is either contraindicated or not initiated. In the United States, federal regulations have existed in some form since 1941, with some of the most significant changes occurring with the passage of the Infant Formula Act of 1980.[5] Monitoring and revisions of federal statues continue to this day under the purview of the US Food and Drug Administration (FDA).

Currently, infant formulas are available in 3 forms: powder, liquid concentrate, and ready-to-feed liquids. Many new parents and guardians have questions regarding local water safety or are unclear about how to safely prepare and use formula. Detailed yet clear information about preparation and storage of infant formula should be made available to the family. An example of such information may be found on the Healthy Children Web site at https://www.healthychildren.org/English/ages-stages/baby/feeding-nutrition/Pages/How-to-Safely-Prepare-Formula-with-Water.aspx.[6]

All infant formulas contain many of the same basic components: proteins, carbohydrates, fats, vitamins and minerals, emulsifiers, and stabilizers, as well as thickeners or diluents. The FDA regulates the ingredients that are deemed necessary in infant formulas along with the minimum and maximum amounts of various nutrients. **Box 1** lists a complete list of nutrients required by the FDA of all manufacturers.[7] Formulas may be exempt from these requirements in certain instances, such as formulas for infants with an inborn error of metabolism, low birth weight, genetic anomalies, or other unusual medical or dietary problems.[8] **Table 1**[9] gives an overview of commonly available types of formula available.

Most formulas are classified into different categories based on their protein source, carbohydrate source, and caloric density.[10] *Caloric density* is commonly 20 calories per ounce in full-term infant formulas but is higher in preterm and transitional formulas.

The *protein source* is commonly cows' milk or soy protein. The main proteins in both human and cows' milk are casein and whey. Whey is digested much more quickly than casein. In human milk, the whey-to-casein ratio is 70:30, whereas in cows' milk it is 18:82.[11] This ratio is modified to 60:40 when developing milk-based human formula

---

Box 1
Nutrients regulated in nonexempt formulas by the US Food and Drug Administration

- Protein

- Fat

- Linoleic acid

- Vitamins
  - Vitamin A
  - Vitamin D
  - Vitamin E
  - Vitamin K
  - Thiamine
  - Riboflavin
  - Vitamin B6
  - Vitamin B12
  - Niacin
  - Folic acid
  - Pantothenic acid
  - Biotin
  - Vitamin C
  - Choline
  - Inositol

- Minerals
  - Calcium
  - Phosphorus
  - Magnesium
  - Iron
  - Zinc
  - Manganese
  - Copper
  - Iodine
  - Sodium
  - Potassium
  - Chloride

From Code of federal regulations title 21. vol. 2. U.S. Food and Drug Administration. 2015. Available at: http://www.accessdata.fda.gov/scripts/cdrh/cfdocs/cfcfr/CFRSearch.cfm?fr=107. 100. Accessed March 1, 2016.

---

in order to more closely mimic breast milk and improve digestibility. When soy protein is used, it is typically supplemented with other amino acids such as L-methionine, L-carnitine, and taurine.[12]

Other important components include the source of *carbohydrate* and the source of fat. Lactose is the key carbohydrate in most cows' milk–based formulas, whereas most soy formulas contain corn syrup solids. Some hypoallergenic or nonallergenic formulas even use sucrose as their source of carbohydrate.[10] *Vegetable oils* are added to formulas in specific blends to mimic the fat content of breast milk.

Vitamins and minerals are also added to all formulas, including iron, calcium, vitamin D, and others. The inclusion of iron deserves particular comment. The AAP recommends that all formula-fed infants receive iron-fortified formula, which typically has 12 mg of iron per liter.[13] "Low-iron" formula has approximately 2 mg of iron per liter. However, there are significant concerns for long-term neurocognitive development following iron deficiency in infancy,[13] and parents should be strongly counseled toward the use of formula with a standard amount of iron.

Table 1
Nutrition options for infants

Milk Type	Examples	Protein	Carbohydrate	Notes
Breast milk	Not applicable	Mixed whey:casein protein ratio	Lactose	The best choice for most babies. Not for mothers with HIV or for infants with galactosemia
Full-term cow's milk–based infant formulas	Enfamil Newborn (Mead Johnson & Co, Glenview, IL, USA), Enfamil Infant (Mead Johnson & Co), Similac Advance (Abbott, Columbus, OH, USA)	Cow's milk protein, varies in whey:casein ratio	Lactose	A common choice for mothers who cannot breastfeed or who choose not to breastfeed
Organic cow's milk–based infant formulas	Similac Advance Organic (Abbott), Earth's Best Organic Infant Formula (Hain Celestial Group, Boulder, CO, USA)	Cow's milk protein, varies in whey:casein ratio	Lactose	Similar to full-term milk-based infant formulas, but for parents with preference for organic products
Cow's milk–based infant formulas with partially hydrolyzed protein	Enfamil Gentlease (Mead Johnson & Co), Gerber Good Start Gentle (Nestle, Florham Park, NJ, USA)	Cow's milk protein, partially hydrolyzed (Goodstart with whey protein only)	Some with lactose, others without	Marketed for "sensitive" babies, but not truly hypoallergenic
Cow's milk–based infant formulas with added thickener	Enfamil Acid Reflux (Mead Johnson & Co), Similac for Spit-Up (Abbott)	Cow's milk protein	Some with lactose, others without; both with added rice starch	Marketed for "spitty" babies

Cow's milk–based infant formulas with little to no lactose	Enfamil Gentlease (Mead Johnson & Co), Similac Sensitive (Abbott), Earth's Best Organic Sensitivity Infant Formula (Hain Celestial Group)	Cow's milk protein: some are partially hydrolyzed, others not	Nonlactose carbohydrates	For babies with galactosemia; marketed for babies with lactose sensitivity or lactase deficiency
Soy formulas	Gerber Good Start Soy (Nestle), Similac Soy Isomil (Abbott)	Soy protein	Nonlactose carbohydrates	For vegan parents, or patients with galactosemia; contains little to no lactose
Preterm infant formulas	Similac Expert Care Neosure (Abbott), Enfamil Enfacare (Mead Johnson & Co)	Cow's milk protein	Lactose	Mixed at 22 kcal/oz
Extensively hydrolyzed cow's milk–based formulas	Nutramigen (Mead Johnson & Co), Pregestamil (Mead Johnson & Co), Similac Expert Care Alimentum (Abbott)	Extensively hydrolyzed milk protein and amino acids	Nonlactose carbohydrates	For cow's milk or soy milk insensitivity. Pregestamil is for patients with steatorrhea
Amino acid–based formulas	Neocate Infant (Nutricia North America, Gaithersburg, MD, USA), EleCare Infant (Abbott)	Amino acids	Nonlactose carbohydrates	For severe protein allergy or short-bowel syndrome

Abbreviation: HIV, human immunodeficiency virus.
From Santiago S. Formula frustrations. Pediatr Ann 2015;44(2):51–4; with permission.

Other additives, although not regulated by the FDA, are used increasingly in infant formulas. These additives include *long-chain polyunsaturated fatty acids (LCPUFAs), prebiotics and probiotics*, and *nucleotides*.

Docosahexaenoic Acid/Arachadonic Acid

Docosahexaenoic acid (DHA) and arachadonic acid (AA) are 2 common LCPUFA added to infant formulas. DHA plays a role in neurogenesis and neurotransmission. Fetal DHA accumulation occurs rapidly during the second half of pregnancy. Studies have correlated a relationship between dietary DHA intake and the DHA concentration in breast milk.[14] As a result, LCPUFA supplementation, particularly DHA supplementation, and its potential benefits have been the subject of intense study.[14,15] Results of several studies have suggested DHA supplementation may promote better vision and improve neurodevelopment, particularly in premature infants.[10,14–18] However, data fail to show statistically significant long-term benefits for term infants who received supplemental DHA.[14] Similarly, analysis of data pertaining specifically to preterm infants failed to find significant results in visual acuity or neurodevelopment.[15] Despite this lack of evidence, most currently available formula preparations now include these fatty acids.

Prebiotics and Probiotics

More recently, formula companies have begun adding prebiotics, probiotics, or a combination of the 2 to formulas. Prebiotics are carbohydrates that cannot be digested by the human body; they are food for probiotics. Probiotics are "good" bacteria that keep your digestive tract healthy by controlling the growth of harmful bacteria. Synbiotics refers to a combination of prebiotics and probiotics.

The goal of these additives is disease prevention, allergy prevention, and the promotion of growth and development. Results of studies have thus far have been inconclusive. A recent systematic review by Mugambi and colleagues[19] evaluated the effects of synbiotics, probiotics, and prebiotics. Although improved weight gain was noted consistently in the study subjects receiving prebiotics, the evidence was not strong enough to suggest improved clinical outcomes with the supplementation of any of the three.

Nucleotides were added to formulas in the late 1990s in an attempt to mimic their high concentration in breast milk, with the understanding that they may have a beneficial effect on growth and the immune system. Although there is some evidence that the addition of these to infant formula may have a positive effect on infant growth,[20] additional research is necessary to ascertain their benefit as a routine formula additive.

FULL-TERM INFANT FORMULAS
Standard Term Formulas

For the healthy term infant who is not breastfed, intact cows' milk protein-based formulas are preferred. The nutrient content of term formula is modeled to match the digestion and absorption of breast milk components.[10,21] These formulas are 20 calories per ounce, which is similar to the caloric load of breast milk, although calories in breast milk can vary slightly. They typically contain lactose as the primary source of carbohydrate, and the source of protein is either intact whey protein or a combination of intact casein and whey from cows' milk.[3,10] These formulas are designed to be nutritionally complete. Common examples of this include Enfamil Premium, Similar Advance, and Parent's Choice Advantage. No one brand is advised to be better than another, including generic brands, and they can typically be used interchangeably.[10]

Infants who have allergies or certain medical conditions may not tolerate standard term infant formulas. A large body of research exists regarding the use of specific infant formulas when neither breast milk nor standard term infant formula is an option. Rare congenital conditions, such as galactosemia and congenital lactase deficiency, as well as more common concerns such as cows' milk protein allergy and lactose intolerance are included. **Table 2**[22,23] reviews differences in presentation between lactose intolerance and cows' milk protein allergy.

Soy Formulas

Although there are a few subtle differences between the compositions of these formulas, the primary feature of all soy formulas includes the fact that they are a milk-free, lactose-free alternative form of complete nutrition to standard term formula. As with standard cows' milk term formulas, soy formulas are also 20 calories per ounce. However, the carbohydrate source is corn based and the protein is isolated from soy. Common examples of these include Enfamil ProSobee, Similac Soy Isomil, and Gerber Good Start Soy.

Soy protein-based formulas attempt to provide adequate nutrition matching both macronutrient and micronutrient composition of cows' milk protein-based formulas.

Table 2
Differentiating between lactose intolerance and cows' milk allergy

	Lactose Intolerance (Lacatase Deficiency)[22]	Cows' Milk Protein Allergy[23]
Age of onset	Typically over age 5	Most common under age 3
Incidence	70% of the world's population, less common among individuals of European descent	2%–3% incidence in first year of life
Gastrointestinal symptoms	Abdominal pain, diarrhea, nausea, flatulence, bloating	Commonly have blood in the stool; diarrhea or constipation; colic and abdominal pain
Respiratory symptoms	None	Rhinorrhea, cough, wheeze, stridor, breathing difficulties
Pathophysiology	Deficiency of lactase, the enzyme required to digest lactose typically found in the small intestine	>50% IgE mediated
Dermatologic symptoms	None	Atopic eczema, urticaria, angioedema
Family history	Hereditary lactose	Atopy, allergic disease common
Other	May be congenital, developmental in preterm infants <34 wk, hereditary, or secondary to small bowel injury, gastroenteritis, or other causes of injury to small intestine mucosa	Failure to thrive, anaphylaxis, metabolic acidosis
Appropriate formula choices	Lactose-free and soy formulas available, but data do not support effectiveness	Soy, amino acid, extensively hydrolyzed formulas

The higher phytate content, however, can interfere with the absorption of minerals, particularly calcium. It is for this reason that soy is not recommended for use in infants born prematurely.[21] Soy formulas are most appropriately used for babies with hereditary lactase deficiency or galactosemia. Soy formulas are also indicated for use in healthy term infants of vegan families wishing to either supplement or replace breastfeeding.

In some cases, parents or caregivers may wish to try a soy formula if an infant shows signs of cows' milk allergy. Studies have suggested cows' milk protein allergy may be as high as 2% to 3% of infants up to 12 months age, with nearly 60% being due to immunoglobulin E (IgE)-mediated intolerance.[24] IgE-mediated reactions typically occur more rapidly than non-IgE-mediated type and can be noted within a couple hours of feeding. Symptoms can include hives, angioedema, abdominal pain, vomiting, diarrhea, and less frequently, rhinorrhea and wheezing.[24]

Infants with IgE-mediated intolerance to cows' milk protein may successfully tolerate soy-based formulas. However, it is important to remember that because of the similarity in protein structure, some infants with milk protein allergy will also have a soy protein allergy.[9] In addition, studies have failed to show a protective effective against later development of food allergies.[24,25]

Lactose Free

Lactose is a disaccharide composed of glucose and galactose found exclusively in mammalian milk. Lactase, the enzyme required for proper metabolism of lactose, is active in various places along the gastrointestinal tract, including the tips of the intestinal villi.[26] Lactase deficiency is commonly referred to as lactose intolerance. It may be primary, which typically fully develops later in childhood; secondary, as a result of small bowel injury; congenital, which is very rare; or developmental, as is typically seen in premature infants.[10,26] Infants experiencing acute episodes of gastroenteritis may develop temporary lactase deficiency.[10] Lactose is a hydrophilic molecule. In the absence of adequate amounts of lactase, lactose will attract fluid and some electrolytes, retaining them in the intestine and therefore increasing the osmotic load of the intestinal contents.[26] Thus, symptoms of lactase deficiency may include abdominal cramping, distention, flatulence, and diarrhea.

Lactose-free formulas are term formulas that use corn syrup solids instead of lactose as a source of carbohydrate.[10] An example of a lactose-free formula is Similac Sensitive; Enfamil Gentlease has a reduced amount of lactose. Soy formulas are also lactose-free.

For infants with galactosemia, primary lactase deficiency, and congenital lactase deficiency, lactose-free formula may be indicated.[10,26] However, lactase deficiency may be overdiagnosed during infancy.[10] During acute gastroenteritis, most infants who were healthy at baseline can safely tolerate remaining on standard term formula versus changing to lactose-free formula. The AAP recommends all breastfed infants continue on human milk throughout an episode of acute gastroenteritis.[26,27] Malnourished infants or formula-fed infants younger than 3 months of age, however, may benefit from temporarily switching to lactose-free formula during diarrheal illness to shorten the duration of gastrointestinal distress.[10,26,27]

Prethickened Formulas

Even for the healthy infant born at term, the lower esophageal sphincter is functionally immature at birth and has decreased tone during the first several months of life.[10] Gastroesophageal reflux (GER) is common among infants, and therefore, is a common cause for parental concern. Prethickened formulas are term infant formulas with added rice starch, also known as antireflux formulas, designed to address this concern.[10,28] Common examples of these formulas include Enfamil AR, Similac Sensitive for Spit-Up, and Parent's Choice Added Rice Starch.

Unless an infant exhibits severe compromise such as weight loss or signs of severe discomfort, GER is not typically treated with medication. Research has shown that infants fed formulas thickened with rice starch had fewer daily episodes of regurgitation and vomiting without impacting gastric emptying.[28]

MODIFIED PROTEIN FORMULAS

If an infant has documented food protein allergy, a hypoallergenic or nonallergenic formula may be appropriate. *Partially hydrolyzed protein formulas* are marketed toward "sensitive" infants. It is important to note that they are not truly hypoallergenic, and there is minimal evidence to support their claims of effectiveness.[29] Examples include Enfamil Gentlease and Gerber Good Start Gentle.

True modified protein formulas include extensively hydrolyzed protein formulas and amino acid–based formulas. *Extensively hydrolyzed protein formulas*, also known as hypoallergenic formulas, have been demonstrated to not cause an allergic reaction in at least 90% of infants with cows' milk allergy. As mentioned previously, more than half of infants with IgE-associated cows' milk protein allergy will experience similar intolerance with soy protein formulas; therefore, a logical next step is to trial hypoallergenic formula.[3,10,24,25] Hypoallergenic formulas are also a useful alternative to breastfeeding for infants with non-IgE-associated intolerances, malabsorption syndromes, and inflammatory syndromes such as proctocolitis, enterocolitis, or esophagitis.[30–32] Common examples of hypoallergenic formulas include Alimentum, Nutramigen, and Pregestimil.

Infants who continue to have symptoms after a 2- to 4-week trial on hypoallergenic formula may require changing to a *nonallergenic free-amino acid–based formula*.[3,10,30] Examples of these formulas include Nutricia Neocate, Abbott Nutrition Elecare, and Enfamil Nutramigen AA. For those infants who require these modified formulas, the AAP recommends continuing either hypoallergenic or nonallergenic formula until 1 year of age or older as needed.[3]

FORMULAS FOR PREMATURE INFANTS
Preterm Formulas

Preterm infant formulas are higher in both protein and calorie concentration. In addition, the content of these formulas has significantly more calcium, phosphorous, and vitamin D to meet the increased metabolic requirements, particularly for those infants born less than 34 weeks gestation or weighing less than 1800 g. Preterm formulas are typically 24 calories per ounce. These formulas are available only for hospital use in ready-to-feed formulations.

Transitional Formulas

Premature infant transitional formulas, also called enriched formulas, are designed to meet the ongoing increased micronutrient and protein demands of the infant born prematurely or small for gestational age.[10] Similar to preterm formulas, these formulas are 22 calories per ounce as well as contain higher amounts of protein, calcium, phosphorous, and vitamin D. Premature transitional formulas include Gerber Good Start Nourish, Enfamil Enfacare, and Similac Neosure. Research suggests improved growth parameters in the short term, but long-term data are inconclusive.[33]

TODDLER FORMULAS

A walk down the aisle of the supermarket will also find a substantial number of toddler formulas, which are marketed toward children from 9 to 24 months of age. These formulas are also milk or soy based and enriched with vitamins, minerals, DHA, and AA. Like infant formulas, toddler formulas are 20 calories per ounce. However, they have slightly greater amounts of proteins and some minerals as compared with standard infant formulas. Although considered nutritionally adequate, families can be counseled that evidence supporting their use is lacking, and their cost is greater than that of milk, in most cases making them a less desirous option.[10] It should be noted that toddler formulas are not the same as pediatric supplemental drinks such as Pediasure and Boost kid Essentials, which are often as high as 30 calories per ounce. Pediatric supplemental drinks are designed to support an already healthy diet for picky eaters, whereas toddler formulas are often an exchange for whole milk for children who continue to consume a primarily liquid diet or who have trouble transitioning to the flavor of regular milk.

ORGANIC FORMULAS

An increasing number of organic infant formulas are available as well. At present, there is no clinical evidence supporting their use. In a 2012 clinical report on organic foods, the AAP specifically noted, "there is no evidence of clinically relevant differences in conventional and organic milk." Clinicians and families may consider both the relatively higher cost of these formulas and the positive environmental impact of using organic formula when weighing this option.[34]

SUMMARY

The AAP and World Health Organization both recommend breastfeeding as the first choice for infant feeding. When breastfeeding is not an option, healthy term infants should be placed on a standard formula unless there is a specific medical indication. Other key points to remember are the following:

- When discussing infant formula with caregivers, care should be taken to obtain a complete history to differentiate between normal infant behavior and true intolerance or allergy.
- Caregivers should be reminded to be skeptical of claims made by formula companies, because many marketing claims have little or no scientific evidence supporting their claims.[29]
- Soy formula is an appropriate first choice for infants with galactosemia and may be tried when there is concern for cows' milk protein allergy.
- Hypoallergenic formula is appropriate for infants with non-IgE-type allergy and malabsorptive syndromes. A change to an amino acid–based formula is appropriate if there is no improvement on the hypoallergenic formula.
- Lactose-free formula may be appropriate for infants with galactosemia, proven lactase deficiency, or high-risk infants with acute diarrhea.
- Antireflux formula may be tried for infants with mild reflux who do not meet criteria for medication. As lower esophageal tone improves with age, however, rechallenging with regular formula after a few months may be appropriate.
- Specialized formulas for preterm infants are available in the hospital, with transition formulas available for premature infants when discharged home.
- Many formulas now contain additives such as LCPUFAs, prebiotics, probiotics, and synbiotics. Although there is no known harm from these products, most

current research also fails to find significant benefit. Additional investigation in these areas is warranted.

REFERENCES

1. Eidelman AI, Schanter RJ, Johnston M, et al. Policy statement: breastfeeding and the use of human milk. Pediatrics 2012;129:e827–41.
2. World Health Organization. Infant and young child feeding: model chapter for textbooks for medical students and allied health professionals. 2009. Available at: http://apps.who.int/iris/bitstream/10665/44117/1/9789241597494_eng.pdf?ua=1&ua=1. Accessed March 2, 2016.
3. Lonnerdal B. Infant formula and infant nutrition: bioactive proteins of human milk and implications for composition of infant formulas. Am J Clin Nutr 2014; 99(Suppl):712S–7S.
4. Breastfeeding among US children born 2002-2012, CDC national immunization surveys. 2015. Available at: http://www.cdc.gov/breastfeeding/data/nis_data/index.htm. Accessed February 27, 2016.
5. United States. Infant formula act of 1980 [report]. Washington, DC: U.S. Govt. Print. Off; 1980.
6. How to safely prepare formula with water. Healthy children web site. 2015. Available at: https://www.healthychildren.org/English/ages-stages/baby/feeding-nutrition/Pages/How-to-Safely-Prepare-Formula-with-Water.aspx. Accessed March 3, 2016.
7. Code of federal regulations title 21, vol. 2. U.S. Food and Drug Administration; 2015. Available at: http://www.accessdata.fda.gov/scripts/cdrh/cfdocs/cfcfr/CFRSearch.cfm?fr=107.100. Accessed March 1, 2016.
8. Draft guidance for industry: exempt infant formula production: current good manufacturing practices (CGMPs), quality control procedures, conduct of audits, and records and reports. U.S. Department of Health and Human Services Food and Drug Administration Center for Food Safety and Applied Nutrition; 2015. Available at: http://www.fda.gov/Food/GuidanceRegulation/GuidanceDocuments RegulatoryInformation/ucm384451.htm. Accessed March 1, 2016.
9. Santiago S. Formula frustrations. Pediatr Ann 2015;44(2):51–4.
10. O'Connor NR. Infant formula. Am Fam Physician 2009;79(7):565–70.
11. Martinez JA, Ballew MP. Infant formulas. Pediatr Rev 2011;32:179–89.
12. Bhatia J, Greek F. Use of soy protein based formulas in infant feeding. Pediatrics 2008;121:1062–8.
13. Baker RD, Greer FR, The Committee on Nutrition. Diagnosis and prevention of iron deficiency and iron-deficiency anemia in infants and young children (0-3 years of age). Pediatrics 2010;126:1040–50.
14. Campoy C, Excolano-Margarit MV, Anjos T, et al. Omega 3 fatty acids on child growth, visual acuity and neurodevelopment. Br J Nutr 2012;107:s85–106.
15. Schulzke SM, Patole SK, Simmer K. Long-chair poloyunsaturated fatty acid supplementation in preterm infants. Cochrane Database Syst Rev 2011;(2):CD000375.
16. Birch EE, Carlson SE, Hoffman DR, et al. The DIAMOND (DHA Intake And Measurement Of Neural Development) study: a double-masked, randomized controlled clinical trial of the maturation of infant visual acuity as a function of the dietary level of docosahexanoic acid. Am J Clin Nutr 2010;91:848–59.
17. Birch EE, Garfield S, Castaneda Y, et al. Visual acuity and cognitive outcomes at 4 years of age in a double-blind, randomized trial of long-chain polyunsaturated fatty acid-supplemented infant formula. Early Hum Dev 2007;83:279–84.

18. Birch EE, Castaneda Y, Wheaton DH, et al. Visual maturation of term infants fed long-chain polyunsaturated fatty acids or control formula for 12 mo. Am J Clin Nutr 2005;81:871–9.
19. Mugambi MN, Musekiwa A, Lombard M, et al. Synbiotics, probiotics or prebiotics in infant formula for full term infants: a systematic review. Nutr J 2012;11:81.
20. Sighal A, Kennedy K, Lanigan J, et al. Dietary nucleotides and early growth in formula-fed infants: a randomized controlled trial. Pediatrics 2010;126:e946–953.
21. De Curtis M, Rigo J. The nutrition of preterm infants. Early Hum Dev 2012;88(1): s1–60.
22. Heyman MB, Committee on Nutrition. Lactose intolerance in infants, children, and adolescents. Pediatrics 2006;118:1279–86.
23. Vandenplas Y, De Greef E, Devreke T. Treatment of cows' milk protein allergy. Pediatr Gastroenterol Hepatol Nutr 2014;17:1–5.
24. Koletzko S, Niggemann B, Arato A, et al. Diagnostic approach and management of cows'-milk protein allergy in infants and children: ESPGHAN GI Committee practical guidelines. J Pediatr Gastroenterol Nutr 2012;55(2):221–9.
25. deSilva D, Geromi M, Halken S, et al. Primary prevention of food allergy in children and adults: systematic review. Allergy 2014;69:581–9.
26. Lasekan JB, Jacobs J, Reisinger KS, et al. Lactose-free milk protein-based infant formula: Impact on growth and gastrointestinal tolerance in infants. Clin Pediatr 2011;50(4):330–7.
27. Heubi J, Karasov R, Reisinger K, et al. Randomized multicenter trial documenting the efficacy and safety of a lactose-free formula for term infants. J Am Diet Assoc 2000;100:212–7.
28. Vandenplas Y, Leluyer B, Cazaubiel M, et al. Double-blind comparative trial with 2 antiregurgitation forumulae. J Pediatr Gastroenterol Nutr 2013;57:389–93.
29. Belamarich MD, Bochner RE, Racine AD. A critical review of the marketing claims of infant formula products in the United States. Clin Pediatr 2016;55(5):437–42.
30. Hill DJ, Murch SH, Rafferty K, et al. Diagnosis and management of cows' milk protein allergy in infants. World J Pediatr 2012;8(1):19–24.
31. Baker SS, Cochran WJ, Frank WJ, et al. Hypoallergenic infant formulas. Committee on Nutrition. Pediatrics 2000;106(2):346–9.
32. Vandenplas Y, DeGreef E, ALLAR study group. Extensive protein hydrolysate formula effectively reduces regurgitation in infants with positive and negative challenge tests for cows' milk allergy. Acta Paediatr 2014;103(6):e243–50.
33. Henderson G, Fahey T, McGuire W. Nutrient-enriched formula versus standard term formula for preterm infants following hospital discharge. Cochrane Database Syst Rev 2012;(4):CD004696.
34. Forman J, Silverstein J, Committee on Nutrition, Council on Environmental Health, American Academy of Pediatrics. Clinical report: organic foods: health and environmental advantages and disadvantages. Pediatrics 2012;130:E1406–15.

Atrial Septal Defects

Kristyn S. Lowery, MPA, PA-C*

KEYWORDS

- Atrial septal defect • Congenital heart disease • Cardiac surgery • Amplatzer
- Ostium secundum • Ostium primum • Sinus venosus • Unroofed coronary sinus

KEY POINTS

- The second most common congenital heart defect is an atrial septal defect (ASD). Patients may be asymptomatic, making thorough examination and diagnostic imaging necessary.
- The secundum ASD is the most common type. Primum, sinus venosus, and unroofed coronary sinus atrial communications may have additional associated cardiac anomalies.
- Percutaneous device closure is possible in secundum ASDs with sufficient surrounding tissue if the device placement does not interfere with other anatomic structures.
- Surgical repair may be performed for all types of ASDs. Mitral valve repair and baffling of a pulmonary vein or left superior vena cava may be executed simultaneously.
- The success rate for closure of ASDs is high. The complication risk is slightly higher in surgical closures; however, both are generally well tolerated.

INCIDENCE AND PREVALENCE

An estimated 1.35 million infants worldwide are born with congenital heart disease every year. This corresponds to approximately 8 in 1000 live births.[1] In the United States, congenital heart defects are the most common birth anomaly, found in 1 of every 100 births and the most common cause of infant mortality.[2] Of all the types of congenital heart disease, ASDs represent the second most common and account for 7% to 10% of all congenital heart defects.[1,3–5] Worldwide, ASDs are noted to be 1.64 per 1000 live births with a female-to-male ratio of 2:1.[3,6]

The most common type of atrial septal communication is an ostium secundum defect, representing 80% of all ASDs. Ostium primum and sinus venosus defects each represent approximately 10%. The rarest type of ASD is an unroofed coronary sinus.[7,8]

EMBRYOLOGY

Commencing 20 days after conception, the cardiovascular system begins to develop. Blood vessels begin to form a tubular heart.[9] This tubular heart constricts into various

Disclosure: The author has nothing to disclose.
Department of Pediatric Cardiothoracic Surgery, Children's Hospital of Pittsburgh of UPMC, 4401 Penn Avenue, Pittsburgh, PA 15224, USA
* Corresponding Author.
E-mail address: Kristyn.Lowery@chp.edu

Physician Assist Clin 1 (2016) 553–562
http://dx.doi.org/10.1016/j.cpha.2016.05.004
2405-7991/16/© 2016 Elsevier Inc. All rights reserved.
physicianassistant.theclinics.com

segments, thereby dividing it from top to bottom into the truncus arteriosus, bulbus cordis, ventricular area, and atrial area. By day 23, the tube begins to loop, resulting in the formation of the primitive heart. The atria then become repositioned within the pericardium as 1 common chamber. The venous drainage localizes to opposite sides of the posterior common atrium. The sinoatrial junction localizes to the right, and the cardinal veins, umbilical vein, and vitelline vein localize to the left side of the common atrium. It is because of these venous junctions that the atria have smooth posterior walls.

At approximately day 35 of gestation, the atrium begins to form 2 separate cavities. It experiences external compression from the truncus arteriosus and the bulbus cordis. Concurrently, the septum primum is developing internally. This is the beginning of the atrial septum. The septum primum has a bowl shape and extends superiorly to the atrioventricular canal and the junction of the mitral and tricuspid valves. The septum secundum then begins to develop to the right of the septum primum. At the end of the process, the only opening that remains is the foramen ovale, which is a slitlike opening between the primum and secundum septums.[5,6] This opening continues to permit blood to flow across the atria during fetal circulation.[9] In certain instances, there is a defect in the wall between the right-sided pulmonary veins and the superior vena cava, which is associated with partial anomalous pulmonary venous return.[8,10]

Several changes occur in the fetal heart when the infant is born. As oxygen enters the lungs, pulmonary vascular resistance decreases. As blood enters the pulmonary vasculature, the afterload for the right ventricle is lowered and left ventricular volume is increased. This change in intracardiac pressure closes the flaplike structure of the patent foramen ovale. The patent ductus arteriosus, which is a vessel that connects the aorta to the pulmonary artery, also contracts and closes after birth. The closure of these communications is necessary for isolating the venous blood to the right side of the heart and pulmonary circulation and the arterial blood to the left side of the heart and systemic circulation.[11]

ANATOMY OF ATRIAL SEPTAL DEFECTS

There are 4 main types of ASDs, including ostium secundum, ostium primum, sinus venosus, and unroofed coronary sinus. As their names indicate, they are differentiated by their location. **Fig. 1** demonstrates the intracardiac location of each of these defects.

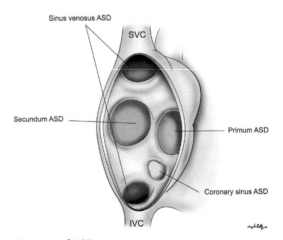

Fig. 1. Intracardiac location of ASDs.

Ostium Secundum Atrial Septal Defect

The morphologic subtype that is the most common ASD is the ostium secundum defect. The communication between the atria is in a central location and caused by a defect in the septum primum. It is typically separate from the vena cavae, pulmonary veins, coronary sinus, and mitral and tricuspid valves. These defects can range in size from 2 mm to 3 cm[6,7,11,12] (**Fig. 2**).

Ostium Primum Atrial Septal Defect

An ostium primum ASD represents approximately 10% of all ASDs. It is the consequence of a septum primum that failed to completely form inferiorly at the junction with the atrioventricular valves. This type of defect is often associated with a cleft in the mitral valve. When this occurs, it is often referred to as a partial atrioventricular septal defect or partial atrioventricular canal. It differs from a complete atrioventricular septal defect due to the lack of a ventricular septal defect and presence of separate mitral and tricuspid valve orifices.[7,11,13]

Sinus Venosus Atrial Septal Defect

A sinus venosus ASD is an opening in the atrial septum near the insertion site of the vena cava into the right atrium. This may happen near the inferior vena cava but is more commonly associated with the superior vena cava. It is often found in conjunction with partial anomalous pulmonary venous return. In most cases, the right upper pulmonary vein is found to enter into the right atria near the entrance of the superior vena cava or directly into the superior vena cava itself. Sinus venous ASDs account for approximately 10% of all ASDs.[6,14,15]

Unroofed Coronary Sinus

The rarest of all ASDs is an unroofed coronary sinus. The coronary sinus drains the venous return from the heart muscle and courses posteriorly in the left atrioventricular groove to terminate into the right atrium. In certain patients, the wall separating the coronary sinus from the left atrium is underdeveloped and the venous blood drains in the left atrium. It then communicates with the right atrium via the septal orifice of the coronary sinus.[7]

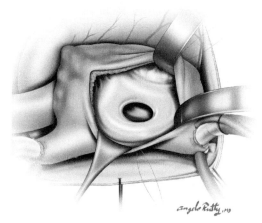

Fig. 2. Intraoperative picture of a secundum ASD.

PHYSIOLOGY

The ratio of pulmonary blood flow to systemic blood flow should be 1:1. This is ratio is referred to as the Q_p:Q_s ratio. Pulmonary vascular resistance is less than systemic vascular resistance; therefore, when there is an opening in the atrial septum, blood shunts from the left to the right causing an increase in the Q_p:Q_s ratio. The amount of shunting is determined by the size of the defect, atrial pressures, and the difference in ventricular compliance between the right and left ventricles. Shunting across the ASD may result in a ratio as great as 4:1.[11] Therefore, the larger the ASD and the worse left ventricular compliance the greater the Q_p:Q_s ratio.

Shunting from right to left across an ASD results in several sequelae. The right ventricular volume is increased causing right ventricular dilatation and hypertrophy. This dilation can force the ventricular septum to bulge to the left, affecting the left ventricle and ultimately causing a decrease in left ventricular function. The right atrium can also become dilated, which can be an impetus for atrial arrhythmias. Over time, increased pulmonary blood flow due to an ASD can cause changes in the pulmonary vasculature resulting in pulmonary hypertension. It has also been shown that paradoxic emboli, or a thrombus from the venous system that crosses to the systemic flow, may occur resulting in a stroke.[6]

DIAGNOSIS

Many children with an ASD may be asymptomatic or only have mild symptoms on exertion, such as tachypnea, shortness of breath, or sinus tachycardia. With larger defects, children may exhibit signs of failure to thrive.[3,12] These symptoms may be easily missed in children. Because of this, the physical examination is relied on for a diagnosis. On auscultation, an increase in pulmonary blood flow results in a systolic ejection murmur best heard on the right upper and middle sternal border. It is typically medium pitched and does not produce a thrill. A fixed split-second heart sound may also be appreciated due to the increase in pulmonary blood flow and the delay in closure of the pulmonary valve. This does not change with inspiration.[7,11,12]

A chest radiograph may show cardiomegaly and increased pulmonary vascular markings. On close examination, an enlarged pulmonary artery may also be visualized on the top left of the cardiac silhouette.

An ECG typically demonstrates normal sinus rhythm, although first-degree atrioventricular block and an rSR[1] can occur. These conduction abnormalities are due to a mild conduction delay through the right ventricle. Right ventricular hypertrophy and right axis deviation arise due to overload of the right ventricle.[7,12]

The most common diagnostic modality for ASDs is a 2-D transthoracic echocardiogram.[6,8] With the use of this diagnostic tool, the location and size of the defect can be determined. Rims surrounding the defect are assessed, which can aid in the decision for the method of closure. With primum ASDs, a cardiologist or sonographer examines the mitral valves for the presence of mitral insufficiency due to a mitral cleft. The echocardiogram may also reveal anomalous drainage of one or more of the pulmonary veins with sinus venosus defects.

The shunt between the atria is viewed using pulsed and color flow Doppler on echocardiography. Cardiologists are able to determine the size and direction of this shunt. A patient may also be suspected to have an ASD if there is an increase in the right ventricular volume with dilatation of the pulmonary artery. Due to right ventricular volume overload, the ventricular septum may be noted to be flattened or move anteriorly during systole instead of posteriorly.[7,8,11,12] These findings clue a cardiologist to look for a septal irregularity and measure the pulmonary arterial pressure. The use of this diagnostic modality has been reported to show 100% of primum ASDs, 89% of secundum ASDs, and 44% of sinus venosus ASDs.[8] The sensitivity of transthoracic echocardiography is greater in children because they have better acoustic windows due to less obesity and an overall smaller body habitus.[6]

If an ASD is suspected, but unconfirmed, a bubble study may be performed during the echocardiogram. This is done by infusing agitated saline through a peripheral intravenous catheter. The patient is then asked to perform a Valsalva maneuver during the echocardiogram. This maneuver causes a temporary right-to-left shunt if a defect is present. It is more easily seen due to the bubbles that cross the defect in the septum.[8]

Cardiac MRI remains the gold standard for depicting ventricular volumes and function. This study can quantify the Qp:Qs ratio to determine the hemodynamic significance of the defect. MRI is also helpful in identifying the anatomy of pulmonary veins when they are sometimes difficult to distinguish on a standard transthoracic echocardiogram. Despite excellent images and information, this study is rarely needed for secundum and primum ASDs.

CT may also diagnose ASDs; however, the exposure to radiation is typically seen as unnecessary due to the sensitivity of echocardiography and MRI.[6]

MANAGEMENT OF ATRIAL SEPTAL DEFECTS

The most significant predictive factor for spontaneous closure of ASDs is size.[16–18] The smaller the communication, the more likely is it to close spontaneously. Studies in 1993 and 2006 found that atrial communications less than 3 mm do not require follow-up because 98.6% of the cases observed closed in 18 to 45 months.[16,18] Other studies report that a defect less than 4 mm will most likely close without intervention.[19] For defects greater than 4 mm, patients need to be followed and monitored for signs of congestive heart failure. The determining factor is the ratio of pulmonary to systemic blood flow. If the $Q_p:Q_s$ is greater than 1.5:1, then patients likely experience right ventricular overload and pulmonary overcirculation. This increase in right-sided volume may be treated medically by diuretics, such as furosemide. Decreasing the afterload with medications like acetylcholinesterase inhibitors may also decrease the degree of shunting through the ASD.[3,17]

An intervention should be performed for closure of the ASD if the patient is symptomatic, has $Q_p:Q_s$ ratio greater than 1.5:1, or has a complication related to the ASD, such as a paradoxic embolism.[11,17,20] The 2 possible methods for closing secundum ASDs are percutaneous closure performed by an interventional cardiologist and surgical closure by a cardiothoracic surgeon. Primum, sinus venosus, and unroofed coronary sinus ASDs all require surgical closure.[4,7] Timing of intervention is typically at 3 to 4 years of age because it is preferable to be done before a child starts school to prevent an interruption education.[3,11,12]

Transcatheter Closure

The first transcatheter closure of a secundum ASD was described by King and Mills in 1976.[5,6,21] This was groundbreaking because it finally created an alternative to surgery. Unfortunately, as the world awaited follow-up on the initial patients, there was little growth in this field until 1983, when William Rashkind reported successful closure of a secundum ASD with a foam-covered, circular device with radiating ribs. The ribs were designed with 3 hooks on the end. This innovation led to the development of the clamshell device by Lock and colleagues.[4,5] The clamshell has been described as a double-hinged paired umbrella with 4 arms that folded on themselves. Unfortunately, clinical trials were stopped due to fracturing of the device and residual shunting. In 1993, the Angel Wing (Microvena Corporation) device was created, which was covered with Dacron (polyethylene terephthalate), using a square design. This was found to have flaws with retrieval and also device erosion. In 1998, a report was published regarding the Amplatzer (AGA medical corporation) septal occluder. This device was made with a nitinol wire mesh, a nickel and titanium alloy, as opposed to foam or Gore-Tex. The waist of the device is the diameter of the ASD and is surrounded on both sides by a disk.[22] These disks are approximately the thickness of the atrial septum. After completion of clinical trials, it was approved by the United States Food and Drug Administration in 2001.[5] In 2006, the Gore Helex occluder was approved by the Food and Drug Administration. It is also made with nitinol wire but is covered with a polytetrafluoroethylene (PTFE) membrane and does not require a long sheath.[23] The Figulla (Occlutech) ASD Occluder is a newer device that has also been used. It is also composed of nitinol wire but has no hub on the left-sided disk.[4,20] Overall, device modifications over the years have made percutaneous closure of ASDs a relatively safe alternative to surgery.

Prior to an attempt of percutaneous closure, the cardiologist must determine the location and size of the ASD. The defect must have adequate rims, or tissue surrounding the defect, to anchor the device. The cardiologist must also ensure that the defect is not located near the systemic or pulmonary venous return or atrioventricular valves.[6] If an ASD seems amenable to percutaneous closure, the patient is brought to the cardiac catheterization laboratory. General anesthesia is typically necessary with pediatric patients.[5] The device is introduced through the femoral vein and deployed within the defect using fluoroscopy and echocardiogram guidance. Heparin is given during the procedure and most institutions prescribe an antiplatelet medication, such as aspirin or clopidogrel after placement.[8] The patient is admitted to the hospital for observation and is typically discharged the following day after an echocardiogram and ECG are performed.[6]

Surgical Repair

In 1939, at Columbia Presbyterian Hospital, the first effort at surgical closure of an ASD was made. This was done by attempting to invert the atrial appendage and use the fascia lata to seal the communication.[4] Twelve years later, Lewis and Tauffic[24] became the first to operate within the human heart when they used hypothermia and clamping the inflow of the heart while suturing an ASD patch in less than 6 minutes. In 1953, after the revolutionary invention of the cardiopulmonary bypass machine, Dr John Gibbon became the first surgeon to close an ASD using cardiopulmonary bypass.[25]

For surgical repair, patients are taken to the operating room and receive general anesthesia. A median sternotomy is made and the thymus is divided or resected. In most cases, a section of the pericardium is harvested for later use. Cardiopulmonary bypass is initiated and cardioplegia is given to stop the heart. An incision is made in the right atrium and the defect can be visualized. For secundum ASDs, the defect may be closed primarily by approximating the sides and closing with sutures. If the defect is large, a patch is used. Pericardium or a synthetic material, such as PTFE or Dacron, may be used as a patch to close the defect (**Fig. 3**).

Primum ASDs are not amenable to primary closure. Prior to closure of a primum ASD, the mitral valve must be evaluated. If a cleft is present, sutures are used for closure to decrease mitral insufficiency. The primum ASD is then typically closed with a pericardial patch.[13]

Sinus venosus ASDs also require patch closure due to the association with partial anomalous venous return. In most cases, the patch is used to baffle the arterial blood

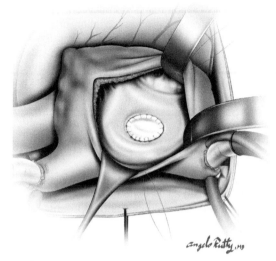

angelo Restly, mg

Fig. 3. Patch closure of a secundum ASD.

to the left atrium while closing the ASD. This can either be done using a 1-patch or 2-patch technique. When the pulmonary vein drains high in the superior vena cava (SVC) or if the surgeon believes that a patch may compromise flow through the SVC, a 2-patch technique or a Warden procedure may be used. In the Warden procedure, the SVC is transected superior to the pulmonary veins and is then reanastomosed to the right of the right atrial appendage.[26]

An unroofed coronary sinus may also be repaired using a pericardial patch. This defect is often associated with a left superior vena cava, which may require baffling, or redirecting, to the right atrium.

After surgical closure of an ASD, the patient is admitted to the ICU and remains in the hospital for a total of 2 to 3 days.[11]

OUTCOMES AND COMPLICATIONS
Device Closure

For secundum ASDs closed via a transcatheter device, a procedural success rate of 93% to 96% with a closure rate of 98% to 99% has been reported.[6] The complication rate is approximately 7%. The initial concern for device closure was the risk of erosion; however, this has only been shown to occur in 0.1% of percutaneous closures. A thorough history prior to placement is important due to the possibility of a nickel allergy reaction. Patients with a nickel allergy due to the nitinol wire device may develop headaches, fever, rash, pericardial effusion, or respiratory symptoms that could necessitate removal of the device and surgical closure of the defect.[4] Arrhythmias may also occur. Atrioventricular block may be more common in children than adults with device closures due to the size of the ASD and device.[27] Atrial arrhythmias, including atrial flutter or atrial fibrillation, may also occur after closure.[28–31] Periprocedural complications may occur but are rare. These include device embolization and pericardial tamponade. Patients may also experience vascular compromise after cardiac catheterization resulting in loss of pulses in the lower extremity and requiring temporary anticoagulation with heparin.[6]

Surgical

As with device closure, surgical repair has a mortality risk nearing 1% and a success rate of approximately 99%; however, the complication profile may be greater than percutaneous closure. Surgical closure requires cardiopulmonary bypass, which carries the risk of stroke. Morbidities, including bleeding, pleural effusions, and arrhythmias, may occur. After ASD repair, patients may also have postoperative pericarditis demonstrated with diffuse ST segment changes on ECG and a friction rub on physical examination. Due to the sternotomy incision, pain is also a factor in the postoperative period. These patients do not require anticoagulation or antiplatelet therapy after surgery.

SUMMARY

Cardiac anomalies are the most common birth defect in the United States. Of all congenital heart defects, ASDs are the second most common. Diagnosis of these defects requires a thorough physical examination and appropriate imaging, because patients may be asymptomatic. Overall, both surgical and percutaneous closures of significant ASDs have an extremely low mortality rate with a survival curve not unlike the general population. Advances in diagnostics, transcatheter device design, and surgical technique allow children with ASDs to live long, healthy lives.

ACKNOWLEDGMENTS

The author would like to extend a special thank you to Dr. Victor Morell for his guidance and education of the past ten years as her collaborating physician and the Chief of Cardiothoracic Surgery at Children's Hospital of Pittsburgh of UPMC. She would also like to thank Angelo Rutty, MD, for the illustrations for this publication.

REFERENCES

1. Van der Linde D, Konings EE, Slager MA, et al. Birth prevalence of congenital heart disease worldwide: a systematic review and meta-analysis. J Am Coll Cardiol 2011;58(21):2241–7.
2. Lee LJ, Lupo PJ. Maternal smoking during pregnancy and the risk of congenital heart defects in offspring: a systemic review and metaanalysis. Pediatr Cardiol 2013;34:398–407.
3. Shuler CO, Tripathi A, Black GB, et al. Prevalence of treatment, risk factors, and management of atrial septal defects in pediatric medicaid cohort. Pediatr Cardiol 2013;34:1723–8.
4. Moore J, Hedge S, El-Said H, et al. Transcatheter device closure of atrial septal defects. JACC Cardiovasc Interv 2013;6(5):433–42.
5. King TD, Mills NL. Secundum atrial septal defects: nonoperative closure during cardiac catheterization. JAMA 1976;235–2506.
6. Geva T, Martins JD, Wald RM. Atrial septal defects. Lancet 2014;383:1921–3.
7. Goldberg SP, Kozik D, Willis C, et al. Atrial septal defects. In: Munoz R, Morell V, da Cruz EM, et al, editors. Critical care of children with heart disease. London: Springer; 2010. p. 159–67.
8. Martin SS, Shapiro EP, Mukherjee M. Atrial septal defest – clinical manifestations, echo assessment, and intervention. Clin Med Insights Cardiol 2014;8:93–8.
9. Abdulla R, Blew GA, Holterman MJ. Cardiovascular embryology. Pediatr Cardiol 2004;25:191–200.

10. Attenhofer Jost CH, Connolly HM, Danielson GK, et al. Sinus venosus atrial septal defect: Long term post-operative outcome for 115 patiens. Circulation 2005;112: 1953–8.

11. Backer CL, Mavroudis C. Atrial septal defect. Partial anomalous pulmonary venous connection, and scimitar syndrome. In: Mavroudis C, Backer CL, editors. Pediatric cardiac surgery. 3rd edition. Philadephia: Mosby; 2003. p. 283–97.

12. Kliegman RM, Stanton BF, St Geme JW, et al. Acyanotic congenital heart disease. In: Kliegman R, Stanton BF, St. Geme JW, et al, editors. Nelson textbook of pediatrics. 20th edition. Philadelphia: Elsevier; 2016. p. 2189–99.

13. Najm HK, Williams WG, Churatanaphong S, et al. Primum atrial septal defect in children: early results, risk factors, and freedom from reoperation. Ann Thorac Surg 1998;66(3):829–35.

14. Agrawal SK, Khanna SK, Tampe D. Sinus venosus atrial septal defect: surgical follow-up. Eur J Cardiothorac Surg 1997;10:456–7.

15. Adatia I, Gittenberger-de Groot AC. Unroofed coronary sinus and coronary sinus orifice atresia: implications for management of complex congenital heart disease. J Am Coll Cardiol 1995;25(4):948–53.

16. Bostan OM, Cil E, Ercan I. The prospective follow-up of the natural course of interatrial communications diagnosed in 847 newborns. Eur Heart J 2007;28: 2001–5.

17. Saito T, Ohta K, Nakayama Y, et al. Natural history of medium-sized atrial septal defects in pediatric cases. J Cardiol 2012;60:248–51.

18. Radzik D, Davignon A, van Doesburg N, et al. Predictuve factors for spontaneous closure of atrial septal defects diagnosed in the first 3 months of life. J Am Coll Cardiol 1993;22(3):851–3.

19. Helgason H, Jonsdottir G. Spontaneous closure of atrial septal defects. Pediatr Cardiol 1999;20(3):195–9.

20. Godart F, Houeijeh A, Recher M, et al. Transcatherter closure of atrial septal defect with the Figulla® ASD occlude: a comparative study with the Amplatzer ® septal occluder. Arch Cardiovasc Dis 2015;108:57–63.

21. Bishnoi RN, Everett AD, Ringel RE, et al. Device closure of secundum atrial septal defects in infants weighing less than 8Kg. Pediatr Cardiol 2014;35:1124–31.

22. Thanopoulos BD, Laskari CV, Tsaousis GS, et al. Closure of atrial septal defects with the Amplazer occlusion device: preliminary results. J Am Coll Cardiol 1998; 31(5):1110–6.

23. Latson LA, Zahn EM, Wilson N. Helex septal occlude for closure of atrial septal defects. Curr Interv Cardiol Rep 2000;2(3):268–73.

24. Lewis FJ, Taufic M. Closure of atrial septal defects with aid of hypothermia: experimental accomplishments and report of one successful case. Surgery 1953;33:52–9.

25. Gibbon JH Jr. Application of a mechanical heat and lung apparatus to cardiac surgery. Minn Med 1954;37(3):171–85.

26. Okonta KE, Tamatey M. Is double or single patch for sinus venosus atrial septal defect repair the better option in prevention of postoperative venous obstruction? Interact Cardiovasc Thorac Surg 2012;15:900–3.

27. Wang Y, Hua Y, Li L, et al. Risk factors and prognosis of atrioventricular block after atrial septum defect closure uring the Amplazer device. Pediatr Cardiol 2014; 35:550–5.

28. Kutty S, Hazeem A, Brown K, et al. Long-term (5- to 20-Year) outcomes after transcatheter or surgical treatment of hemodynamically significant isolated secundum atrial septal defect. Am J Cardiol 2012;109:1348–52.

29. Ates AH, Sunman H, Aytemir K, et al. Prevention of recurrent crytogenic stroke with percutaneous closure of patent foramen ovale; one year follow-up study with magnetic resonance imaging and holter monititoring. Turk Kardiyol Dern Ars 2015;43(1):38–46.
30. Yilmazer MM, Güven B, Vupa- Çilengiroğlu Ö, et al. Improvement in cardiac structure and functions early after transcatheter closure of secundum atrial septal defect in children and adolescents. Turk J Pediatr 2013;55:401–10.
31. Hoffman J, Kaplan S. The incidence of congenital heart disease. J Am Coll Cardiol 2002;39(12):1890–900.

An Overview of Pediatric Asthma

Brian R. Wingrove, MHS, PA-C, DFAAPA

KEYWORDS

- Asthma • Pediatrics • Inhaled corticosteroids • Spirometry

KEY POINTS

- Asthma is a chronic inflammatory disorder of the airways that causes recurrent episodes of respiratory symptoms, particularly at night or in the early morning. These episodes are often reversible spontaneously or with treatment.
- Inhaled steroids should be used as controller therapy in children who have asthma exacerbations.
- Spirometry should be used as a tool for diagnosing asthma and for monitoring response to therapy.
- Asthma can be treated early and aggressively with bronchodilators, and oral steroids should be made available at home for at-risk patients.

INTRODUCTION

Approximately 7 million children in the United States have asthma, accounting for 9.3% of those under the age of 18 years. It is estimated that the prevalence of disease is around 16% for African American children, 9% for Hispanic children, and up to 25% of inner city children. It is more common in boys than in girls until adolescence.[1] This chronic illness causes a significant level of morbidity, including 14 million missed school days and 200,000 hospitalizations per year, and in 2013, accounted for 183 deaths among children aged 14 years and under.[2,3]

The National Heart, Lung, and Blood Institute (NHLBI) released guidelines for the diagnosis and management of asthma in 2007. A random sample of 829 pediatricians revealed a self-reported adherence rate of only 39% to 53% to the previously released guidelines in 1997. Unfortunately, provider adherence to the NHLBI guidelines remains low. Reasons given for nonadherence include a lack of confidence in following the guidelines, lack of outcomes expectancy, and a lack of time, resources, and staff.[4] Given asthma's prevalence and burden, strategies for improving confidence and

Disclosure Statement: The author has nothing to disclose.
Children's Physician Group–Pulmonology, Scottish Rite, Children's Healthcare of Atlanta, 1100 Lake Hearn Drive, Suite 450, Atlanta, GA 30342, USA
E-mail address: brian.wingrove@choa.org

Physician Assist Clin 1 (2016) 563–582
http://dx.doi.org/10.1016/j.cpha.2016.05.005

resource utilization would be important for improving outcomes in asthma management.

WHAT IS ASTHMA?
Pathophysiology

Asthma is defined by the NHLBI as a chronic inflammatory disorder of the airways that causes recurrent episodes of wheezing, breathlessness, chest tightness, and coughing. These episodes are often reversible either spontaneously or with treatment.[5] Pathophysiologically, asthma is identified by the triad of airway edema, constriction of the bronchial tubes, and excess mucus production. Inflammation is mediated by many cellular elements, including neutrophils, eosinophils, mast cells, leukotrienes, T lymphocytes, and epithelial cells. Together these 3 elements contribute to the hyperresponsiveness, airflow limitation, and airway obstruction, leading to the characteristic symptoms of asthma (**Fig. 1**).

Symptoms

Wheezing is produced by a vibration in the airways as airflow is obstructed by a narrowed segment of the bronchial tree. It is more common during the expiratory phase of breathing because increased intrathoracic pressures result in increased compression of the bronchioles. Wheezing is high pitched and biphasic. As air moves through a compressed segment of an airway, the flow becomes turbulent, causing vibration of airway walls; the pitch of the wheeze changes as air travels proximally from small bronchioles to the larger, more central airways.

Although wheezing is often considered the hallmark symptom of asthma, cough is frequently the presenting symptom. Cough is the most common chief complaint in the United States and Australia.[6] Although the differential diagnosis of cough in children is extensive, asthma is by far the most common cause of a chronic or recurrent cough. A diagnosis of asthma should always be entertained in any child with recurrent cough. A cough at night is the most common type of asthma cough.[7] A cough first thing in the morning and a cough with exercise are also very characteristic of asthma (**Fig. 2**).

An asthma cough may be wet, dry, or mixed. Bronchospasm occurs when a deep inhalation provokes coughing fits (3 or more coughs in a row). These coughing fits are

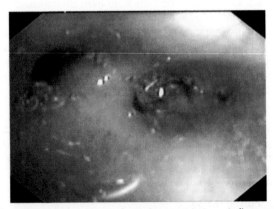

Fig. 1. Pathologic features of asthma: bronchoconstriction, inflammation, and mucus production.

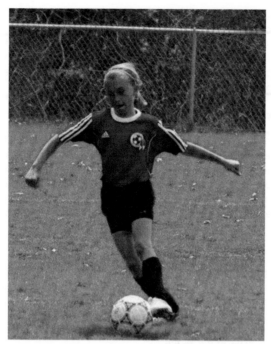

Fig. 2. A cough with exercise or play, at night time, or first thing in the morning is characteristic of asthma.

characterized by spasms of rapid succession coughing that can make administration of inhaled medications difficult. There can often be a vibratory quality to the cough even if a wheeze is not audible. In these cases, the cough is frequently dry, although excess mucus production is part of the pathophysiology of asthma so the cough can become "wet."

Shortness of breath results as air trapping occurs in obstructed bronchial tubes leading to an inability to adequately inhale to a full vital capacity, or to exhale fully. This same air trapping leads to the sensation of chest tightness and pain.

Expression

Three phenotypes of asthma have been identified.[7] The first cohort is children presenting early in life with wheezing primarily with viral upper respiratory infections. These episodes of wheezing recur with less frequency over time and mostly resolve by the preschool years. A second group is those with a later onset of symptoms, typically after the age of 3 years with persistence into adolescence. The final group identified had early onset of obstructive symptoms that persisted throughout childhood. The final group had confirmed atopy, the degree of which did not differ from the late-onset wheezers. All 3 groups showed lower expiratory flows, forced expiratory volume in 1 second (FEV1), and FEV1/forced vital capacity (FVC) ratio than those children who had never wheezed.[7]

Childhood asthma has the potential to persist and to relapse. Of 613 New Zealand children followed from ages 9 years to 26 years, 27.4% had remission of their asthma symptoms over time, but of those, 12.4% had relapsed.[7] Even those children with transient wheezing showed reduced airway caliber by 6 years of age, with increasing evidence that airway remodeling can occur at young ages.[7] Despite this, asthma remains underdiagnosed and undertreated. A study of 122,829 children in North Carolina public schools aged 12 to 14 years showed that 17% of them reported asthma symptoms but had never been diagnosed with asthma. Of those 17%, there was significant reported morbidity with 20% missing school; 25% with limitations to activity; 32% having sleep disturbance; 7% with Emergency Department treatment; and 5% with hospitalization.[8]

DIAGNOSING ASTHMA

One of the challenges in diagnosing asthma involves separating the precipitating factor from the disease itself. Rhinovirus has been implicated as a major precipitant of airway inflammation, and respiratory viruses in general have been isolated in about 80% of childhood asthma exacerbations.[9] It is important to recognize that the diagnosis of a viral respiratory infection does not preclude the diagnosis of asthma. Clinicians should assess risk factors for underlying abnormality in addition to treatment of the acute illness.

Risk Factors

Establishing a diagnosis of asthma can be facilitated by the use of a predictive index.[3] The index criteria used in association with a history of 3 episodes of wheezing in 12 months, or 2 episodes requiring systemic corticosteroids in 6 months, provide a 77% specificity for diagnosing asthma. The risk factors are seen in **Table 1**.

The presence of one major factor, or any 2 of the minor factors, raises the risk of asthma by an odds ratio of 2.6 to 5.5.[7]

The Third National Health and Nutrition Examination Survey performed a cross-sectional analysis of 12,380 children from 1988 to 1994.[10] This analysis revealed an odds ratio for having asthma of 4.00 if there was a parental history of asthma or hay fever; a ratio of 1.94 in those with a body mass index greater than 85%; and a ratio of 1.64 in those of African American ethnicity (**Table 2**).

Pulmonary function testing of FVC, FEV1, and mid-expiratory flow rate (FEF 25%–75%) is a useful tool for assessing airway obstruction.[11] It is particularly useful if there is positive response to administration of a bronchodilator. Spirometry in children presents unique challenges but can be achieved with success in children over the age of 5 years with personnel experienced in administering the test to children (**Fig. 3**).

Spirometry provides an objective assessment of control, helps identify obstruction in those with low symptom awareness, allows the clinician to track disease progression, and helps measure response to therapy.[5] Spirometry is performed by having the child inhale deeply to near total lung capacity and then forcefully exhale into the spirometer as hard and fast as they can to near residual volume. It requires the child to seal their lips on the mouthpiece and to wear a clip to prevent air escaping through the nose. Visual cues, like the bowling scenario in the photograph in **Fig. 3**, to aid the child in focusing on achieving a goal are helpful to improve the validity of testing. The

Table 1 Asthma risk factors	
Major	**Minor**
Atopic dermatitis	Allergic rhinitis/aeroallergen sensitivity
	Wheezing without colds
Parental history of asthma	Eosinophilia on nasal smear or blood count

Table 2
Identification of population subgroups

Odds Ratio 4.00	Odds Ratio 1.94	Odds Ratio 1.64
Parental history of asthma or hay fever	Body mass index >85%	African American ethnicity

test is repeated 3 times to prove reproducibility. The computer measures the volume and rate of air exhaled into the device and calculates percentages based on predicted values. The predicted values are based on gender, height, and ethnicity. Achievement of 80% of the predicted value is considered normal, below that is obstruction, particularly any disproportionate reduction in the FEV1 to the FVC. A bronchodilator should then be administered, and the test repeated, looking for a statistically significant change of 12% or more in the FVC, FEV1, and the FEV1/FVC ratio. There is conflicting evidence about the amount of change required to be statistically significant in the FEF 25% to 75%. A positive bronchodilator response is highly suggestive of asthma as it is evidence of reversible airway obstruction (**Table 3**).

ASSESSING ASTHMA
Severity

Once a diagnosis of asthma has been made, a clinician should further determine the level of severity to aid in guiding therapeutic interventions. There are 2 components included to determine severity: risk and impairment. Risk is the utilization of emergent health care interventions. To assess risk, a patient or caregiver should be asked to enumerate visits to emergency rooms (ERs) or urgent care centers, and if any of those visits resulted in hospitalization. Particular attention should be paid to any admission to an intensive care unit (ICU) or respiratory failure requiring endotracheal intubation.

Impairment seeks to evaluate the frequency of symptoms and the use of bronchodilators for relief, and the impact those symptoms have on play or exercise, sleep, and school attendance. A symptom frequency of greater than 2 of any of the following indicates persistent asthma:

- Days per week
- Nights per month
- Days of albuterol used per week
- Exacerbations in 6 months

Current guidelines classify asthma as mild, moderate, or severe depending on the frequency of symptoms, the presence of night-time symptoms, and lung function. The severity of the asthma classification is based on the worst variable (**Table 4**).

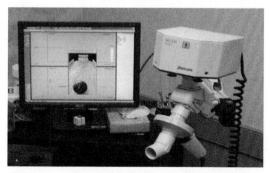

Fig. 3. Spirometry.

Table 3
Spirometry showing obstructed forced expiratory volume in 1 second, forced expiratory volume in 1 second/forced vital capacity ratio, and forced expiratory flow 25% to 75% with a statistically significant reversibility after use of a bronchodilator

	Pred	Pre	% Pred	Post	% Pred	% Change
FVC [L]	2.04	2.02	99.0	2.22	108.8	10.0
FEV1 [L]	1.83	1.44	78.7	1.91	104.3	32.5
FEV1% FVC [%]	—	71.29	—	85.91	—	20.5
FEF 25–75 [L/s]	2.24	1.01	45.3	2.01	89.8	98.4

Abbreviations: Pre, before bronchodilator administration; Pred, predicted.

Control

The Asthma Control Test (ACT) is a validated questionnaire that is reliable for assessing asthma control.[12] The ACT is written for children of 2 different age groups: those ages 4 to 11 years, and those over the age of 12 years. The patient or caregivers answer each question with a point rating; a low score indicates poorly controlled asthma (**Boxes 1** and **2**).

Peak flow monitoring offers clinicians a means for monitoring asthma. Peak expiratory flow rate, or peak flow for short, measures the maximal rate that a person can exhale during a short maximal expiratory effort after a full inspiration. Peak flows are measured and recorded at home, but adherence drops off considerably. The efficacy of peak flow monitoring has not been consistent in various studies, and the advantage of peak flows over symptom monitoring has not been demonstrated.[13]

Spirometry differs from peak flow monitoring in measuring volume versus rate. Spirometry has the advantage over peak flow because it is done under the supervision of a trained health care professional who can provide coaching and detect manipulation or less than adequate effort. Spirometry is recommended in the NHLBI guidelines for diagnosing asthma, assessing response to therapy, evaluating patients during a period of loss of control of asthma symptoms, and repeating annually for surveillance.

MEDICATIONS
Bronchodilators

Many patients with mild asthma do not require daily controller medications, but should have access to short-acting β-agonists (SABAs) to use when symptoms are present.

Table 4
Asthma classification based on severity and symptoms

Severity	Symptoms	Night-Time Symptoms	Lung Function
Severe persistent	Continual symptoms Limited physical activity Frequent exacerbations	Frequent	FEV1 <60%
Moderate persistent	Daily symptoms Daily use of bronchodilators Exacerbations >2/wk	>1/wk	FEV1 >60% but <80%
Mild persistent	Symptoms >2/wk but <1/d Exacerbations may affect activity	>2/mo	FEV1 >80%
Mild intermittent	Symptoms <2/wk Asymptomatic between exacerbations	<2/mo	FEV1 >80%

Box 1
Asthma control test questionnaire (ages 4–11)

ACT: ages 4 to 11

1. How is your asthma today?

2. How much of a problem is your asthma when you run, exercise, or play sports?

3. Do you cough because of your asthma?

4. Do you wake up during the night because of your asthma?

5. During the last 4 weeks, on average, how many days per month did your child have any daytime asthma symptoms?

6. During the last 4 weeks, on average, how many days per month did your child wheeze during the day because of asthma?

7. During the last 4 weeks, on average, how many days per month did your child wake up during the night because of asthma?

The SABAs are bronchodilators that are fast acting on β-2 receptors in the airway to induce smooth muscle relaxation and enhance ciliary beat frequency, thereby improving air flow. The β-2 agonists include albuterol, levalbuterol, and pirbuterol and are available in metered dose inhalers (MDIs) and as nebulized solutions.

Inhaled Corticosteroids

If asthma is determined to be persistent, then starting a daily controller medication should be strongly considered. Inhaled corticosteroids (ICS) are the most effective medication for controlling asthma.[14] They increase pulmonary function, reduce the risk of severe asthma-related outcomes, and reduce the need for additional medication use. In the United States, there are 6 available ICS that come in 3 types of delivery devices: nebulized (budesonide), MDIs (fluticasone, beclomethasone, ciclesonide, mometasone, flunisolide), and dry powder inhalers (DPIs; fluticasone, mometasone, budesonide). The dosage of these medications varies, but a reasonable strategy is to start by dosing twice daily using 1 vial of the nebulized medication, 2 puffs of the MDIs, or 1 inhalation of the DPIs. Patients with more mild asthma can be managed with lower doses of ICS, but those with more persistent or severe symptoms should be started on high dose. The doses are not necessarily based on age, but on the

---

Box 2
Asthma control test questionnaire (ages 12 and up)

ACT: ages 12 and up

1. In the past 4 weeks, how much of the time did your asthma keep you from getting as much done at work, school, or home?

2. During the past 4 weeks, how often have you had shortness of breath?

3. During the past 4 weeks, how often did your asthma symptoms wake you up at night or earlier than usual in the morning?

4. During the past 4 weeks, how often have you used your rescue inhaler or nebulizer medication?

5. How would you rate your asthma control during the past 4 weeks?

severity of asthma. One reasonable strategy is to start with a moderate dose of ICS to get control quickly and prove that the medications work, then step down at follow-up (**Table 5**).

Nebulized medication is the least efficient delivery system.[15] Although simple to use, nebulization is the most time consuming of the 3 delivery modalities, taking up to 20 minutes depending on the device in use (**Fig. 4**). Delivery is achieved through simple tidal breathing of the aerosolized medication with a mask firmly secured to the face. Attempting blow-by administration, with the mask removed from the face, decreases delivery efficiency profoundly and should not be done. A common misconception is that crying increases deposition of the medication into the airways. Air movement while crying can be characterized by a long (often loud) expiratory phase with a short staccato inspiratory phase. In fact, this will further decrease the amount of medication deposited.

MDIs show a greater degree of airway deposition than nebulizers. They are faster to use and more easily portable. With MDIs, however, it is essential to use a spacing device. Medication is dispensed from the MDI canister with ejection velocities estimated in the range of 150 to 225 m per second. Scintigraphy studies have demonstrated decreased oropharyngeal deposition with use of a spacing device leading to improved asthma control.[15] Spacers increase the amount of medication deposited into the lung by 3-fold by increasing the fine particle size of the droplets, thus decreasing the amount of nonbreathable medication.[16] In addition, by using a spacer and decreasing the oropharyngeal deposition, the side effect of candidiasis can be dramatically reduced. For all these reasons, all children, regardless of age, should be encouraged to use a spacer (**Fig. 5**).

Spacers come in a variety of types with subtle variations, but typically come with either a mask or a mouthpiece. With masked devices, it is important to ensure a good fit from the bridge of the nose to the chin, especially as a child grows. Masked devices are easy to use and generally well tolerated by young children. They, like nebulizers, rely on tidal breathing until a child is old enough to be coached to take deep breaths. Proper technique involves the following:

- Placing the mask to the child's face
- Shaking the MDI device vigorously and inserting into the spacer
- Activating the canister with a single pump
- Watching for 6 to 10 tidal breaths, or have child inhale deeply if able to do so
- Repeating actuations as prescribed/indicated

Mouthpiece devices require inspiratory force sufficient to atomize the medication and inhale it into the lower airways (**Fig. 6**). Proper technique with this device involves the following:

- Shake the MDI device vigorously and insert into the spacer
- Exhale fully

Table 5 Inhaled corticosteroids		
Nebulized	**MDI**	**DPI**
Budesonide (Pulmicort)	Fluticasone (Flovent) Mometasone (Asmanex) Beclomethasone (Qvar) Ciclesonide (Alvesco) Flunisolide (Aerospan)	Fluticasone (Flovent) Mometasone (Asmanex) Budesonide (Pulmicort)

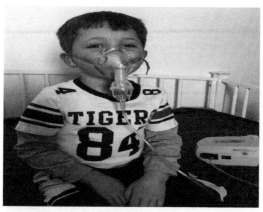

Fig. 4. Nebulized medication.

- Enclose lips around the mouthpiece
- Actuate canister with a single pump
- Inhale slowly and deeply
- Remove spacer and hold breath for 5 to 10 seconds
- Repeat actuations as prescribed/indicated

Technique is crucial with this device and should be checked at every visit. Although superior to using a masked spacer, it must be done correctly to be effective. The inhalation should focus more on inspiring a large volume versus a rapid rate of the breath. Many spacers have a whistle built into the device to signal if the rate of the breath is too rapid to be effective.

DPIs are the newest delivery devices. The steroid molecule is not suspended in a solution and so may have more direct interaction with the lung epithelium. Although reported to have greater potency, there is no difference in the efficacy of DPIs and an MDI with spacer; however, notably, both are superior to an MDI alone. The DPIs do not require a spacing device and are the most easily portable of all the devices.

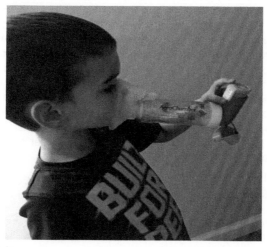

Fig. 5. Spacing device.

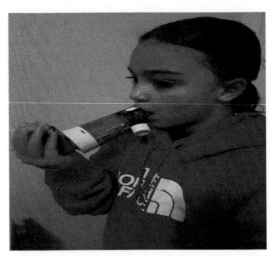

Fig. 6. Mouthpiece device.

Technique is paramount and should be reviewed at every visit. It is quite similar to the use of the mouthpiece spacer, except the rate needs to be faster in order to pull the medication out of the DPI device and atomize it.

The most common side effect of the ICS drugs is thrush, followed closely by dysphonia.[17] Side effects can be avoided by rinsing out the mouth and brushing the teeth after use of ICS. Another consideration is the possibility of growth suppression. However, this risk is considered small and should be weighed against the importance of gaining asthma control and reducing exacerbations. In a study of the burden of ICS, 285 children aged 2 to 3 years were assigned to fluticasone propionate (FP) 88 μg twice per day with a spacer or placebo for a 2-year treatment period and then were observed without treatment for 1 additional year.[17] There was significant improvement in symptom-free days for those in the FP group with more episode-free days, decreased exacerbations, and decreased need for extra medication. Those in the ICS group did show a 1.1-cm decrement in growth after the first 2 years of the study, but this difference decreased to 0.7 cm after the 1-year observation period. A different study of adults who had been treated with the ICS budesonide as children were, on average, about half an inch shorter than their counterparts who were not treated with ICS. The half-inch difference had been observed when the study participants were children, showing that, although the effect on height may persist through adulthood, the overall change is minimal.[18]

Although there is limited evidence about superiority or inferiority of one device over another, population studies do not reflect differences between individuals. There are also no data about whether patient preference influences adherence. What works best is what the patient will use and use correctly. Consider the following factors when choosing an ICS for patients:

- Age of the child
- Severity of disease
- Cognitive level of the child and of the caregiver
- Willingness to use the device
- Time commitment, portability
- Insurance coverage/cost

There are no differences in cost between the various delivery modalities (nebulized vs MDI vs DPI), depending on the patient's insurance formulary. Most insurances have preferred medications in each class.

Leukotriene Receptor Antagonists

Leukotrienes are potent inflammatory mediators produced in many cells. Various stimuli may activate their release or activation. One leukotriene in particular, LTD4, is one of the most powerful bronchoconstricting agents. Leukotriene receptor antagonists (LTRAs) block leukotrienes from binding to their receptors in the inflammatory cascade. LTRAs decrease activation of eosinophils and the release of cytokines. Montelukast has been shown to be the most efficacious of these medications with the most favorable safety profile.[19]

Although ICS are the gold-standard medication for asthma controller therapy, montelukast is considered an alternative monotherapy in mild asthma, especially as part of a step-down strategy. ICS are more effective than LTRAs, but when montelukast is added to an ICS, studies have shown further improvement in pulmonary function and in symptomatic control.[20] The addition of montelukast may also result in an ability to reduce the dose of ICS. However, only 15% of patients show a greater response to montelukast than to ICS.[19]

When compared with the addition of a long-acting β-agonist (LABA), results have been inconclusive. Short-term studies indicated a lower rate of exacerbations for those on montelukast versus on an LABA. Longer-term studies showed the 2 treatments were similarly effective at reducing exacerbations.[19] Given the heterogeneous nature of asthma, it is recommended to tailor therapy based on individual response. LTRAs seem to be most effective in the following types of asthmatics[19]:

- Asthmatics with exercise-induced asthma
- Asthmatics with asthma associated with allergic rhinitis
- Obese patients
- Asthmatics with viral-induced wheezing

Long-Acting β-Agonists

Another option for add-on therapy when a single-agent ICS is insufficient to control asthma is the LABAs. The LABAs are essentially long-acting bronchodilators that exert their relaxation of smooth muscle for 12 hours. They are not fast acting and should not be used for quick relief of asthma symptoms. LABAs should never be used as a single agent in children. They must always be used with an ICS, as a combination, never as separate agents. There are 3 commercially available ICS/LABA products: mometasone/formoterol (Dulera); budesonide/formoterol (Symbicort); and fluticasone/salmeterol (Advair). Fluticasone/salmeterol is available as an MDI and a DPI; mometasone/formoterol and budesonide/formoterol are only available as an MDI.

The 2006 release of data from The Salmeterol Multicenter Asthma Research Trial Study showed a statistically significant increase in asthma-related deaths in those receiving salmeterol.[21] Because of the results of this study, all 3 combination medications carry a US Food and Drug Administration (FDA)-mandated Black Box warning. This outcome is contrary to numerous other studies showing a benefit of an ICS/LABA combination therapy.[22,23] The cause of the increased deaths remains unclear, although it has been postulated that there are genetic and ethnic differences in the expression of asthma among African Americans as well as an overall lack of use of ICS at baseline in the study. Once asthma control is achieved on a combination medication, consideration should be made to step down to a single agent as soon as possible without losing control.

ADJUSTING THERAPY
Stepping Up

After initiating medical therapy for controlling asthma, if symptoms are inadequately controlled, it is advised to increase therapy. A simple way to do this is to increase the dose of the steroid and is the preferred first step.[5] The other alternative is to add a second medication like an LTRA or to switch to an ICS/LABA combination medication. It can be difficult to know which medication will induce the best response. A clinician should also gauge the effect on adherence that adding a second medication will have versus using a combination medication, which may still be perceived as only one drug. The following tables are meant to aid the clinician in decision making, but ultimately it is the response of the individual that must be closely monitored.

Adding LTRA	Adding LABA
Under age 12 y	Over age 12 y
Intermittent symptoms	Daily or persistent symptoms
Allergic rhinitis	Frequent symptoms with exercise
Snoring/upper airway obstruction	Frequent bronchodilator use

Before making any changes to the medication regimen, however, it is essential to assess adherence and technique. A poster with the various inhalers in full color is helpful when speaking with some families.

- Identify the medication; make sure there is differentiation between the controller and the rescue medication.
- How is it used (once or twice a day, 1 puff or 2)?
- How often do you forget to use it?
- Is the child supervised? Reminded? Doing it solo?
- Is a spacer is being used with MDIs?
- How well is the toddler or young child tolerating having a mask on their face?
- Demonstrate technique with the delivery device (MDI/spacer or DPI).

If there are deficiencies in any of these areas, concentrate on improving those aspects that can be modified before increasing the medication burden.

Stepping Down

Control of asthma can be defined as a lack of impairment with minimal symptoms, and a reduction in risk of having a significant exacerbation. Once control has been achieved, it is advised to monitor for a minimum of 3 months to ensure clinical stability. It is recommended, in particular, to monitor through a season change to ensure that control is not lost with temperature changes (heat or cold) or exposure to the aeroallergens specific to different seasons (trees in spring, grass in summer, weeds in autumn).

Stepping down can be achieved in multiple ways, as follows:

- Reduce the dose of medication
- Reduce the frequency of medication
- Discontinue a medication, if on multiple drugs

Caregiver or patient preference should be considered as well as associated costs of medication and family dynamics. Ultimately, the goal of asthma therapy should be the use of the least amount of medication to maintain the same level of control. With any step down in therapy, families should be given specific guidelines for contacting the health care provider to report failure, and interventions should there be breakthrough symptoms. Close follow-up is necessary to ensure continued stability with no decline in lung function.

Stepping-up and stepping-down therapy can be a constant, moving target. Young children tend to do very well during the spring and summer months when there are fewer circulating respiratory viruses and can be stepped down; however, with the arrival of the cold and flu season, therapy is likely going to need to be stepped back up. Follow-up is always crucial to gauge response to therapy and to work with families in maintaining good control of asthma.

ALLERGY MANAGEMENT

For any patient with persistent asthma, an evaluation of the role of aeroallergens, particularly indoor precipitants, is recommended.[5] Identification of allergic triggers can aid the caregiver and patient to avoid exposures by taking steps at interventions if possible and can direct medical therapy.[24] Skin testing is considered the gold standard for allergy testing. There is no age limitation, but in young children, particularly younger than 6 months, there has been insufficient exposure to develop sensitization to allergens. Reactivity to skin testing in the very young is lessened, and fewer tests can be performed due to a smaller body surface area. Under the age of 4 years, children are more likely to be sensitized to indoor allergens such as dust mites, cockroaches, mold, and pet dander. Not until after the age of 4 years would a child typically demonstrate sensitization to outdoor pollens.

Once specific aeroallergen triggers have been identified, a multifaceted approach to avoidance and reduction of exposure should be planned. Consider immunotherapy in those in whom there is a strong correlation between symptoms and a positive reaction to an allergen.

Some patients may still have poorly controlled asthma despite use of multiple medications and appropriate avoidance strategies. Omalizumab is a humanized monoclonal antibody that targets immunoglobulin E (IgE) receptors on mast cells and basophils, preventing binding of IgE. These cells are downregulated and their activation is inhibited, as is the subsequent release of their inflammatory mediators.[25] Omalizumab has been shown to reduce asthma exacerbations and the frequency of ER visits and hospitalizations. It also improves symptomatic control and overall quality of life. Some studies have indicated an ability to decrease both oral and ICS use. A US study showed clinically relevant improvements in asthma control, which were maintained during 2 years of longitudinal follow-up.[26]

Omalizumab is indicated down to the age of 12 years for the treatment of severe persistent allergic asthma that remains uncontrolled with frequent exacerbations, despite high-dose combination therapy, and documented sensitization to a perennial aeroallergen and an IgE level of 30 to 700 (based on recommended dosing schedules). Omalizumab is an injection given every 2 weeks or every 4 weeks depending on the IgE level. Omalizumab carries a risk of anaphylaxis and so should be administered only in a medical facility with personnel equipped to respond to an anaphylactic emergency. It is recommended to observe patients for a minimum of 2 hours after the first injection, and for 30 minutes with subsequent injections.[25]

MANAGING EXACERBATIONS

Asthma has the potential to worsen and cause episodes of increasing symptoms when a patient is exposed to inciting triggers. Caregivers and patients should always be counseled to avoid exposure to provoking aeroallergens, avoid tobacco smoke and other respiratory irritants, avoid strenuous outdoor activity when air pollution levels are high, and receive annual influenza vaccination.[5] Pretreatment with a bronchodilator is recommended in situations when avoidance is not possible.

An acute asthma exacerbation is characterized by a reduction in expiratory flow leading to cough, wheezing, shortness of breath, dyspnea, chest tightness, and tachypnea. A child may present with evidence of increased work of breathing with head bobbing, nasal flaring, or retractions of the suprasternal, intercostals, or subcostal muscles. Severe air trapping and mucus production may lead to atelectasis; auscultation of the lungs may demonstrate decreased or absent breath sounds as a result (**Fig. 7**).

Severity of an exacerbation can be mild, moderate, severe, or life threatening. Clinicians and families must be never underestimate the severity of an exacerbation. Any exacerbation can become life threatening regardless of the severity of the underlying asthma. Certain factors have been identified for those at high risk of a fatal asthma attack[5]:

- Previous intubation for asthma
- Previous ICU admission for asthma
- Two or more hospitalizations in the past year
- Three or more ER visits in the past year
- Hospitalization or ER visit in the past month
- Use of more than 2 bronchodilator inhalers in a month
- Low socioeconomic status
- Inner city residence
- Illicit drug use
- Psychosocial or psychiatric comorbidity
- No asthma action plan at home

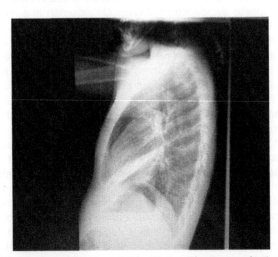

Fig. 7. Right middle lobe atelectasis in a child with an asthma exacerbation. Also evident on this film is hyperexpansion consistent with air trapping.

In mild exacerbations, children may experience dyspnea or cough only with activity. Lung function is generally well preserved or decreased only slightly. These children experience prompt relief with bronchodilator use, although repeat administration may be necessary. Oral corticosteroids are generally not needed, and symptoms last 1 to 2 days.

When symptoms interfere with activity, the exacerbation is considered moderate. These children may require an office or ER visit due to frequent use of bronchodilators. Oral corticosteroids are likely to be needed to abort the exacerbation and improve lung function.

In a severe exacerbation, asthma symptoms occur even at rest. Dyspnea becomes severe enough to interfere with conversation. Only partial relief with bronchodilators is achieved. Oral steroids are necessary, and at times adjunctive therapies may be helpful to enhance bronchodilation. Hospitalization is likely if symptoms cannot be relieved.

Tachypnea and hypoxemia can occur with any degree of severity. Mucus plugging and narrowed airways lead to a ventilation-perfusion mismatch and an inability to deliver oxygen to the alveolar capillary bed. In a mild exacerbation, hypoxemia can be overcome with delivery of a bronchodilator and coughing, thereby enhancing air flow to the distal bronchioles. In more severe exacerbations, the obstruction can be significant enough that hypoxemia will persist until inflammation and bronchoconstriction can be relieved.

As the distress becomes more progressive, a child will begin to tire, and some may experience a sense of impending doom. Oxygenation and ventilation begin to fail as hypercarbia leads to a respiratory acidosis. There is little to no relief with bronchodilators. Intravenous corticosteroids and adjunctive therapies become necessary to sustain life.

Early intervention in an asthma exacerbation is crucial. Caregivers and older patients should be counseled on asthma warning signs and how to intervene. All patients, regardless of their asthma severity, should have a written asthma management plan in place with specific guidelines on medications to be used, quantity and frequency of dosing, and when to seek emergent care **(Fig. 8)**.[27]

Components of an Asthma Management Plan

- Daily controller medications
- What to do when having symptoms like coughing, wheezing, or chest tightness
- What to do if your fast-acting medication is not working
- Identification of triggers

Bronchodilators

Acutely, the first-line treatment for asthma is the use of fast-acting bronchodilators via nebulization or MDI. There is no difference between nebulized or MDI administration, if administered technically correctly.[28] In addition to the bronchodilators discussed in the previous section on medications, ipratropium bromide is another fast-acting bronchodilator. It is an anticholinergic with a more modest bronchodilator effect through relaxing smooth muscle; it also acts as a drying agent, which may help with excess mucus production. Used in combination with β-2 agonists, Ipratropium bromide improves lung function and decreases hospitalization. Used alone, however, treatment failure is more likely.

Frequency is dependent on severity but is typically every 3 to 4 hours in mild disease. Patients may be able to do a repeated cycle of treatments successively to quickly gain control and then resume every 3-hour administration. The author's

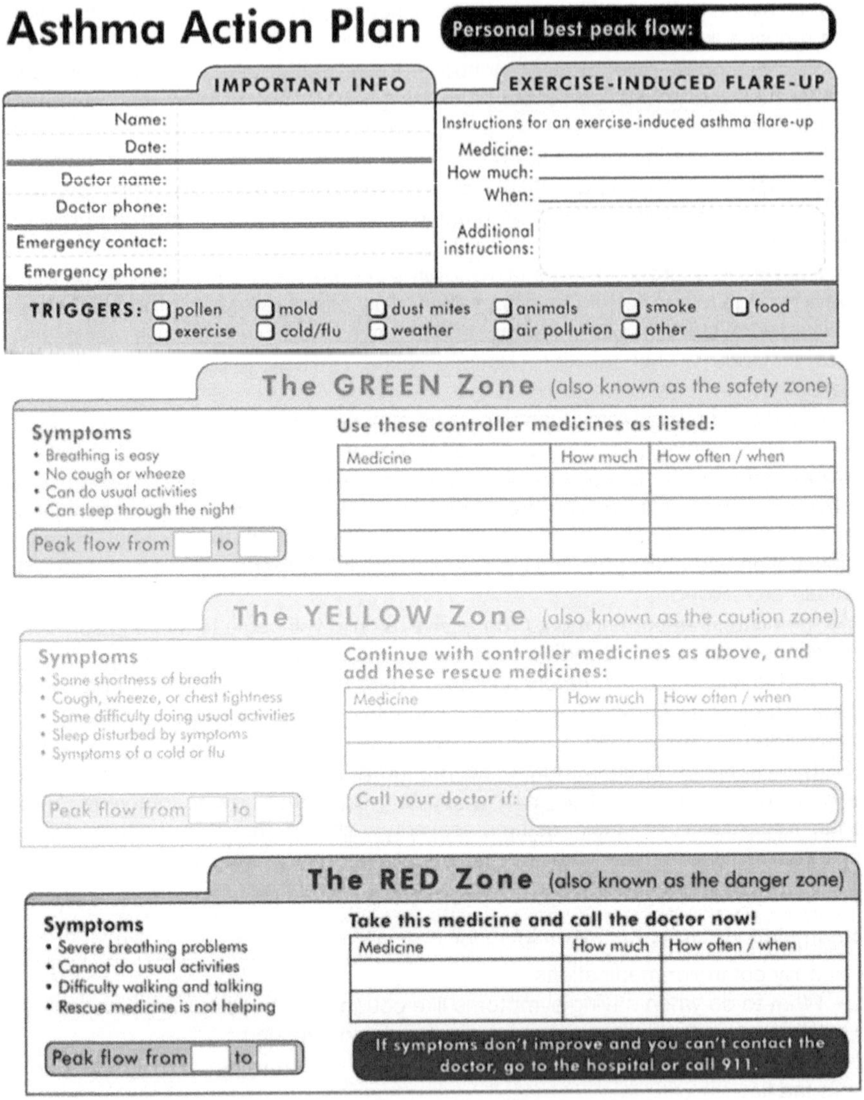

Asthma Action Plan

Personal best peak flow: _____

IMPORTANT INFO

Name: _____
Date: _____
Doctor name: _____
Doctor phone: _____
Emergency contact: _____
Emergency phone: _____

EXERCISE-INDUCED FLARE-UP

Instructions for an exercise-induced asthma flare-up
Medicine: _____
How much: _____
When: _____
Additional instructions:

TRIGGERS: ☐ pollen ☐ mold ☐ dust mites ☐ animals ☐ smoke ☐ food
☐ exercise ☐ cold/flu ☐ weather ☐ air pollution ☐ other _____

The GREEN Zone (also known as the safety zone)

Symptoms
- Breathing is easy
- No cough or wheeze
- Can do usual activities
- Can sleep through the night

Peak flow from ____ to ____

Use these controller medicines as listed:

Medicine	How much	How often / when

The YELLOW Zone (also known as the caution zone)

Symptoms
- Some shortness of breath
- Cough, wheeze, or chest tightness
- Some difficulty doing usual activities
- Sleep disturbed by symptoms
- Symptoms of a cold or flu

Peak flow from ____ to ____

Continue with controller medicines as above, and add these rescue medicines:

Medicine	How much	How often / when

Call your doctor if: _____

The RED Zone (also known as the danger zone)

Symptoms
- Severe breathing problems
- Cannot do usual activities
- Difficulty walking and talking
- Rescue medicine is not helping

Peak flow from ____ to ____

Take this medicine and call the doctor now!

Medicine	How much	How often / when

If symptoms don't improve and you can't contact the doctor, go to the hospital or call 911.

Fig. 8. Asthma action plan.

practice uses a "back-to-back-to-back" cycle where the patient may do a treatment every 20 minutes for an hour, but then must contact the provider on call. In the emergency and hospital setting, continuous bronchodilators are given.

Steroids

When bronchodilators are insufficient to abort asthma symptoms, the next step is to use systemic steroids either orally or parenterally. Intravenous methylprednisolone may be necessary in severe exacerbations or respiratory failure; however, there is no difference in the efficacy of the intravenous versus oral route for steroids.[29] Access to steroids should be part of every asthma management plan, including having a supply at home particularly for severe asthmatics with explicit instructions to contact their health care provider when used.[5]

Studies indicate that short bursts with dexamethasone have been used successfully in place of longer courses of prednisolone.[30] There were favorable differences in vomiting and adherence in the dexamethasone group with no change in outcomes.[29] Prednisolone should be dosed at 2 mg/kg/d to a maximum of 60 mg/d, although higher doses have been used. A typical course is 5 days, although as few as 3 days may be used in milder exacerbations, whereas 10 days may be needed in more severe flares. Dexamethasone is given once daily for 2 days at a dose of 0.6 mg/kg/d to a maximum of 16 mg. If symptoms are still present, switch to prednisolone for continued dosing.

Oxygen

Early administration of supplemental oxygen is recommended in asthma exacerbations. American Heart Association guidelines suggest keeping oxygen saturation greater than 94% in an exacerbation. Oxygen can be used to deliver bronchodilators while also serving to reverse hypoxemia. There are several delivery systems with varying concentrations of delivered oxygen (Fio_2), including low- and high-flow nasal cannulas, simple mask, Venturi mask, partial non-rebreather, and non-rebreather mask. The non-rebreather mask has the capacity to deliver the highest concentration of oxygen up to an Fio_2 of 1.0.[31]

Adjunctive Therapies

Adjunctive therapies for the emergent treatment of acute asthma include magnesium sulfate, terbutaline, and Heliox.

Magnesium sulfate is delivered intravenously and induces smooth muscle relaxation at the bronchial level. Utilization increases lung function and decreases hospitalization rates. It can be given as a single dose of 25 to 100 mg/kg in theER, or repeated every 6 hours if hospitalization is required. A child can be safely discharged from the ER after magnesium sulfate delivery if asthma symptoms improve and blood pressure is stable.

Terbutaline is another intravenous medication used in refractory asthma exacerbations. It is selective for β-2 adrenergic receptors and affects bronchodilation through smooth muscle relaxation. It is a fast-acting agent given in doses of 0.25 mg and can be repeated every 15 to 30 minutes. It is not FDA approved in children under age of 12 years.

Heliox is a low-density gas mixture of oxygen and helium. It has no bronchodilator effect but reduces airway resistance by producing laminar flow in constricted airways where the flow of traditional air mixture is turbulent. The laminar airflow improves the work of breathing and enhances ventilation. There is a lack of concrete evidence on the efficacy of use of Heliox in asthma exacerbations, but further study is warranted.[32]

Ventilatory Support

In a child in whom efforts to affect bronchodilation have failed and whose requirement for substantial amounts of supplemental oxygen remains high, noninvasive positive pressure ventilation can be a useful tool to improve respiratory status. Bilevel positive airway pressure (BiPAP) or continuous positive airway pressure (CPAP) delivered by mask aids in recruiting atelectatic alveoli and thus improves oxygenation and ventilation. Some children may require anxiolytics or sedation to tolerate BiPAP/CPAP.

When a child is no longer able to maintain adequate respiratory effort in the setting of respiratory acidosis, endotracheal intubation and mechanical ventilation become necessary. These children generally require higher pressure settings to stent open constricted airways, with shorter inspiratory times to allow for a longer exhalation. Once oxygenation improves, and ventilation is normalized, settings can be weaned toward extubation.

Any child who requires noninvasive or invasive ventilatory support should be considered at high risk for future life-threatening exacerbations.

Hospital Discharge

Children who require hospitalization for their asthma are at significant risk for future exacerbations. Caregivers of these children should attend an asthma education class with a formalized program taught by a certified asthma educator.[27] Strong consideration should be given to starting these children on ICS given their high risk. Even the provider in the ER plays a role in starting ICS. A small study in New York involved children aged 2 to 18 years of age who presented to the ER with an asthma exacerbation. They were identified by questionnaire as having persistent asthma, and if not already on a controller medication, were given a 2-week supply of an ICS. Of those started on ICS, 70% followed up with the primary care provider, and 75% of those were continued on the ICS.[33]

SPECIALIST CONSULTATION

Pediatric allergists and pediatric pulmonologists are specially trained to treat asthma, its comorbidities, and complications. Indications for referral to an asthma specialist include the following:

- For purposes of obtaining spirometry if unable to do so in the primary care setting
- Patients requiring combination of therapies to maintain control, especially those under the age of 4 years
- Patients with frequent exacerbations and hospitalizations
- Patients who may benefit from immunotherapy or omalizumab if unable to do so in the primary care setting
- Patients in whom the diagnosis is not clear

SUMMARY

Asthma is a chronic disease with significant impacts on a child's quality of life, with the potential for severe adverse outcomes. It requires an individualized approach within evidenced-based guidelines for the diagnosis and management of this disease. Most importantly, early intervention with daily controller medication in the form of ICSs is a standard of care. Guidelines can assist in stepping-up therapy in those who lack control, and stepping-down therapy in those who have attained control of their asthma symptoms. Spirometry is an essential tool in this process. Exacerbations should be anticipated and families prepared with an asthma management plan. Early intervention with bronchodilators is essential, using systemic steroids when the flare cannot be aborted. Hospitalization and intubation are significant risk factors for future life-threatening asthma exacerbations, and these children should be followed closely.

REFERENCES

1. Summary Health Statistics for U.S. Children: National Health Interview Survey 2012. US Department of Health and Human Services, Centers for Disease Control and Prevention. Vital Health Stat 2013;10(258):4.
2. Xu J, Murphy SL, Kochanek KD, et al. Deaths: final data for 2013. Natl Vital Stat Rep 2016;64(2):1–119.

3. Pediatric Asthma: Current Perspectives on Individualized Treatment to Optimize Patient Care. A CME Monograph from Vindico Medical Education. December 2011.

4. Cabana M, Rand CS, Becher OJ, et al. Reasons for pediatrician nonadherence to asthma guidelines. Arch Pediatr Adolesc Med 2001;155:1057–62.

5. Expert panel report 3: guidelines for the diagnosis and management of asthma (EPR-3). National Heart, Lungs, and Blood Institute; US Department of Health and Human Services; 2007. Available at: www.nhlbi.nih.gov/files/docs/guidelines/asthgdln.pdf.

6. ACCP Policy Statement on Cough Management. Chest 2007;129(1):1S–23S.

7. Pohunek P. Pediatric asthma: how significant it is for the whole life? Paediatr Respir Rev 2006;7S:S68–9.

8. Yeatts K, Shy C, Sotir M, et al. Health consequences for children with undiagnosed asthma-like symptoms. Arch Pediatr Adolesc Med 2003;157(6):540–4.

9. Friedlander SL, Busse WW. The role of rhinovirus in asthma exacerbations. J Allergy Clin Immunol 2005;116(2):267–73.

10. Rodriguez M, Winkleby MA, Ahn D, et al. Identification of population subgroups of children and adolescents with high asthma prevalence. Arch Pediatr Adolesc Med 2002;156(3):269–75.

11. McCarthy K. Pulmonary function testing. Medscape 2011. Available at: www.emedicine.medscape.com/article/303239-overview.

12. Schatz M, Sorkness CA, Li JT, et al. Asthma control test: reliability, validity, and responsiveness in patients not previously followed by asthma specialists. J Allergy Clin Immunol 2006;117(3):549–56.

13. Bailey W, Mangan J. Peak expiratory flow rate monitoring in asthma. Up To Date. Available at: www.uptodate.com/contents/peak-expiratory-flow-monitoring-in-asthma.

14. Yoshihara S. Early intervention for infantile and childhood asthma. Expert Rev Clin Immunol 2010;6(2):247–55.

15. Newman S, Newhouse M. Effect of add-on devices for aerosol drug deliver: deposition studies and clinical aspects. J Aerosol Med 2009;9(1):55–70.

16. Corveth H, Kanner R. Optimizing deposition of aerosolized drug in the lung: a review. MedGenMed 1999;1(3). Available at: www.medscape.com/viewarticle/717395_4.

17. Guilber TW, Morgan WJ, Zeiger RS, et al. Long-term inhaled corticosteroids in preschool children at high risk for asthma. N Engl J Med 2006;354:1985–97.

18. Agertoft L, Pedersen S. Effect of long-term treatment with inhaled budesonide on adult height in children with asthma. N Engl J Med 2000;343(15):1064–9.

19. Paggiaro P, Bacci E. Montelukast in asthma: a review of its efficacy and place in asthma therapy. Ther Adv Chronic Dis 2011;2(1):47–56.

20. Vaquerizo MJ, Casan P, Castillo J, et al. Effect of montelukast added to inhaled budesonide on control of mild to moderate asthma. Thorax 2003;58:204–10.

21. Nelson H, Weiss ST, Bleecker ER, et al. The salmeterol multicenter asthma research trial: a comparison of usual pharmacotherapy for asthma or usual pharmacotherapy plus salmeterol. Chest 2006;129:15–26.

22. Bell A, McIvor R. The SMART study. Can Fam Physician 2007;53(4):687–8.

23. O'Byrne PM, Bisgaard H, Godard PP, et al. Budesonide/formoterol combination therapy as both maintenance and reliever medication in asthma. Am J Respir Crit Care Med 2005;171:129–36.

24. Lasley M, Shapiro G. Testing for allergy. Pediatr Rev 2000;21(2):39–43.

25. Holgate S, Buhl R, Bousquet J, et al. The use of omalizumab in the treatment of severe allergic asthma: a clinical experience update. Respir Med 2009;103: 1098–113.
26. Eisner M, Zazzali JL, Miller MK, et al. Longitudinal changes in asthma control with omalizumab: 2-year interim data from the EXCELS Study. J Asthma 2012;49(6): 642–8.
27. Gibson PG, Coughlan J, Wilson AJ, et al. Limited (information only) patient education programs for adults with asthma. Cochrane Database Syst Rev 2000;(2):CD001005.
28. Kajosaari M, Laurikaihen K, Juntunen-Backman K, et al. Comparison of easyhaler metered-dose, dry powder inhaler and a pressurised metered-dose inhaler plus spacer in the treatment of asthma in children. Clin Drug Investig 2002;22(12). Available at: www.medscape.com/viewarticle/446869.
29. Shefrin A, Goldman R. Use of dexamethasone and prednisone in acute asthma exacerbations in pediatric patients. Can Fam Physician 2009;55:704–6.
30. Qureshi F, Zaritshky A, Poirier M. Comparative efficacy of oral dexamethasone versus oral prednisolone in acute pediatric asthma. J Pediatr 2001;139(1):20–6.
31. Chameides L, Samson R, Schexnayder S, et al. Pediatric advanced life support provider manual. American Heart Association; 2011.
32. Reuben AD, Harris AR. Heliox for asthma in the emergency department: a review of the literature. Emerg Med J 2004;21:131–5.
33. Lehman H, Lillis KA, Shaha SH, et al. Initiation of maintenance antiinflammatory medication in asthmatic children in a pediatric emergency department. Pediatrics 2006;118(6):2394–401.

Common Neuromuscular Disorders in Pediatrics

Heather R. Gilbreath, MPAS, PA-C[a,b]

KEYWORDS

- Pediatric neuromuscular disease • Duchenne muscular dystrophy
- Spinal muscular atrophy • Myotonic dystrophy

KEY POINTS

- Duchenne muscular dystrophy (DMD) is an X-linked disorder that affects 1 in 3600 to 6000 live male births. It is due to mutations in the dystrophin-encoding *DMD* gene and is the most common muscular dystrophy.
- Spinal muscular atrophy (SMA) is an autosomal recessive disorder characterized by degeneration of anterior horn cells in the spinal cord and motor neurons in the brainstem. It is due to mutations in the survival motor neuron (*SMN*) gene. Four forms of the disease are recognized in pediatrics.
- Myotonic dystrophy type 1 (DM1) is an autosomal dominant, multisystem disease arising from mutations in the dystrophia myotonica protein kinase (*DMPK*) gene. There are 5 phenotypes of DM1, including congenital myotonic dystrophy (CDM) and childhood-onset myotonic dystrophy.

 Video content accompanies this article at http://www.physicianassistant. theclinics.com.

INTRODUCTION

Neuromuscular disease is a term used to describe rare acquired or inherited conditions that affect a part of the neuromuscular system comprised of anterior horn cells, peripheral motor and sensory nerves, the neuromuscular junction and muscles. The Muscular Dystrophy Association estimates that neuromuscular diseases affect more than 1 million people in the Unites States; approximately 40% of patients are under the age of 18.

All neuromuscular diseases result in varying degrees of muscle weakness and/or muscle fatigue and may present at birth or in childhood or may manifest in adulthood. Life expectancy varies by disease and severity. Neuromuscular diseases are

Disclosure Statement: The author has nothing to disclose.

[a] Children's Health, 1935 Medical District Drive, Dallas, TX 75235, USA; [b] UTSouthwestern Medical Center, School of Health Professions, 5323 Harry Hines Boulevard, Dallas, TX 75390, USA

E-mail address: heather.gilbreath@childrens.com

Physician Assist Clin 1 (2016) 583–597
http://dx.doi.org/10.1016/j.cpha.2016.05.002
2405-7991/16/$ – see front matter © 2016 Elsevier Inc. All rights reserved.

commonly associated with an increased risk of cardiac, respiratory, gastrointestinal, and orthopedic comorbidities, directly related to the effects of muscle deterioration.

Pediatric patients identified as having a neuromuscular disease often present with a history of nonspecific concerns, including hypotonia, developmental delay, and/or muscle weakness. Differential diagnosis can become somewhat of an odyssey for the pediatric provider. Early identification has become essential, given advances in treatment and research opportunities. This article discusses the pathophysiology, diagnosis, and management of 3 common pediatric neuromuscular disorders: DMD, SMA, and myotonic dystrophy.

DUCHENNE MUSCULAR DYSTROPHY
Overview

DMD is an X-linked disorder that affects 1 in 3600 to 6000 live male births.[1] DMD is the most common muscular dystrophy[2] and occurs as a result of mutations in the dystrophin-encoding *DMD* gene. The *DMD* gene is the largest known human gene, containing 79 exons spanning 2.2. Mb. The mutation rate is high, with approximately one-third of cases caused by de novo mutations.[3] Mutations in this gene ultimately lead to an absence of or defect in the dystrophin protein; resulting in either Duchenne or Becker Muscular Dystrophy. This discussion will focus on DMD. Abnormal dystrophin causes progressive muscle degeneration and subsequent muscle weakness. Dystrophin is expressed in skeletal, cardiac, and smooth muscle tissues. Additionally, dystrophin isoforms are expressed in the human central nervous system (CNS).[4] Phenotypic expression can be variable and is directly related to the type of mutation and its effect on the production of dystrophin. Approximately 10% of female carriers show some disease manifestations that may include abnormal cognitive and/or cardiac function.[5]

Clinical Presentation

Patients often present between the ages of 3 and 5 years with a history of mild to moderate delay of motor milestones and progressive muscle degeneration. Parents may cite specific concerns, including frequent falls, difficulty arising from the floor, difficulty climbing stairs, or the inability to run. A history of muscle pain or muscle cramping is commonly associated with the disease as well. A referral to a neurologist or neuromuscular specialist is indicated with these concerns.

On other occasions, patients present to the gastroenterology clinic after identification of persistently elevated aspartate aminotransferase (AST) and alanine aminotransferase (ALT). Although transaminases are typically markers of hepatocellular injury, they are also highly concentrated in muscle cells. The finding of an elevated AST/ALT in the absence of other laboratory abnormalities or clinical concerns associated with hepatic disease warrants further investigation of muscle disease.

Lastly, patients may present secondary to neurobehavioral concerns. Recent literature suggests that 27% of patients have a full-scale IQ of less than 70; 44% have a learning disability; 19% suffer from intellectual disability; 32% struggle with attention-deficit/hyperactivity disorder; 15% carry a secondary diagnosis of autism spectrum disorder; and 27% of patients suffer from anxiety.[4] These concerns, combined with a history of motor delay and/or muscle weakness, deserve further evaluation.

Physical Examination

On examination, patients are found to be mildly to moderately hypotonic with an increase in muscle bulk most commonly in the calves (**Fig. 1**) or in the form of

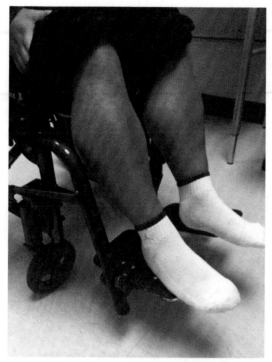

Fig. 1. Calf hypertrophy in a patient with DMD.

macroglossia. Patients suffer from varying degrees of symmetric muscle weakness at presentation but with proximal musculature and lower extremities affected first. Patients most commonly have a Gower sign (**Fig. 2**), standing with the aid of hands pushing off on the knees. Gait deviations may include a wide base with exaggerated lumbar lordosis and waddling. With time, a decreased heel strike is also seen secondary to increasingly tight heel cords. Deep tendon reflexes are typically decreased or absent.

Diagnostic Testing

Initial diagnostic testing for DMD includes a total creatine phosphokinase, also known as a creatine kinase (CK) test. Results yield values of up to 100 times the upper limit of normal. Next steps include DNA analysis of the dystrophin gene. A majority of patients have a deletion or duplication of 1 or more exons. Therefore, it is most cost and labor efficient to check for these mutations first using multiplex ligation-dependent probe amplification (MLPA) analysis. If this testing is negative, providers may proceed with Sanger sequencing of individual exons. In rare cases, a biopsy may be required in patients with a clear DMD phenotype but with no identifiable mutation in the gene. A muscle biopsy uses immunohistochemistry and/or Western blot analysis to determine if dystrophin is absent or present. If absent, additional RNA studies may be performed of the dystrophin gene.[3] If present in normal quantity, it is likely that the patient is suffering from an alternate form of muscular dystrophy.

Progression/Prognosis

Patients diagnosed with DMD suffer from progressive muscle weakness with a steady decline in strength between 6 and 11 years of age. Loss of ambulation is common

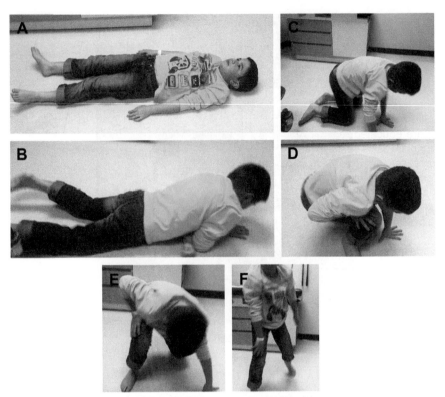

Fig. 2. (*A–F*) Serial images of a Gower sign in a patient with DMD.

between 9 and 13 years of age.[6] Patients develop significant joint contractures with time, secondary to the imbalance of strength in muscle groups. Additionally, scoliosis may develop, typically after the loss of ambulation. Dysphagia and constipation also occur as a result of muscle weakness. Patients eventually suffer from pulmonary complications, including an ineffective cough, nocturnal hypoventilation, sleep-disordered breathing, and ultimately daytime respiratory failure. Dilated cardiomyopathy occurs most commonly in adolescence. Life expectancy is most common between 15 and 25 years of age but can be prolonged with proper respiratory support and/or cardiac interventions.[6]

Treatment Options

Patients with DMD require multidisciplinary care as the disease advances. In addition to neurology, patients are regularly followed by pulmonology, cardiology, and orthopedic specialists. Additionally, patients require ongoing evaluations from physical, occupational, and speech therapists as well as registered dieticians.

The current standard of care for patients with DMD includes the use of glucocorticoids beginning between 3 and 5 years of age. Glucocorticoids have demonstrated the ability to slow the rate of muscle weakness and loss of function in boys with DMD, thereby reducing the risk of scoliosis and stabilizing pulmonary function. Cardiac function may also improve as a result of the use of glucocorticoids. Prednisone, at a dose of 0.75 mg/kg/d, or deflazacort, at a dose of 0.9 mg/kg/d, is the current recommended regimen although alternative dosing strategies exist. Side effects frequently occur and patients must be regularly monitored and managed accordingly.[7]

Patients with DMD should be seen by a pulmonary specialist at the time of diagnosis for a baseline evaluation and regularly thereafter. Pulmonary function testing is completed on an annual basis, specifically measuring the forced vital capacity, peak cough flow, maximal inspiratory/expiratory pressures, and end-tidal CO_2. When forced vital capacity decreases to less than 60% predicted, annual sleep studies are recommended to screen for sleep-disordered breathing. Patients and families are educated regarding manually and mechanically assisted cough techniques and noninvasive ventilation, initially at night and then during the day as the disease progresses. Assisted ventilation via tracheostomy may be considered as a last resort to prolong survival.[8]

Patients with DMD are also regularly followed by a cardiologist. Baseline assessment should be completed at diagnosis and at least once every 2 years until the age of 10. Annual cardiac assessments should begin at 10 years of age or at the onset of cardiac signs and symptoms if they occur earlier. Minimum assessment should include an electrocardiogram and a noninvasive echocardiogram. Evidence supports the treatment of cardiomyopathy associated with DMD before signs of abnormal functioning. Angiotensin-converting enzyme inhibitors are considered first-line therapy.[8]

Patients with DMD are commonly referred to orthopedic specialists secondary to progressive joint contractures and the risk for scoliosis. Monitoring for scoliosis should be regularly performed during clinical observations while the patient remains ambulatory. Spinal radiography is indicated 1 year after the loss of ambulation and annually thereafter.[8] Spinal surgeries may be warranted.

Multiple other specialties assist in the management and care of patients with DMD when needed. Gastroenterologists often treat refractory gastroesophageal reflux and/or severe constipation. Furthermore, endocrinologists regularly assist in the management of bone health and the treatment of growth deficiency when merited.

Patients with DMD are also regularly followed by physical, occupational, and speech therapists. This team of services is vital to ensuring that patients are able to maintain function to the best of their ability, despite progressive muscle weakness. Multiple strategies are utilized, including home programs promoting passive and active range of motion and stretching, orthoses to prevent joint contractures, appropriate use of wheelchairs and other durable medical equipment, and feeding strategies to minimize the effects of dysphagia. Registered dieticians are also an important member of the health care team because patients are commonly either malnourished as a result of dysphagia or are overweight, subsequent to the effects of glucocorticoids and inability to effectively burn calories with exercise due to physical limitations.

Research

Years of research has been aimed at understanding the exact causes of muscle dysfunction in DMD and to apply that understanding to the development of effective treatments. Research strategies currently used include exon-skipping with antisense oligonucleotides (AONs), gene therapy, myostatin inhibitors, and utrophin up-regulators, among others.

SPINAL MUSCULAR ATROPHY
Overview

SMA is an autosomal recessive disorder characterized by degeneration of motor neurons in the anterior horn of the spinal cord and brainstem, resulting in progressive muscular atrophy and weakness.[9] The incidence of the disorder is approximately 1 in 10,000 live births,[10] and it is reported to be the leading genetic cause of infant death.[11] Carrier frequencies are estimated to be 1 in 50.[10] The disorder is caused by mutations within the *SMN* gene, which is responsible for the production of the SMN protein essential to motor neurons. In SMA, insufficient levels of the SMN protein lead to degeneration of the lower motor neurons, producing weakness and wasting of the skeletal muscles.

There are 2 almost identical *SMN* genes present in humans, known as *SMN1* and *SMN2*. *SMN1* is considered the active gene for SMN protein production and more than 98% of patients with SMA have a homozygous deletion in both *SMN1* genes. The *SMN2* gene does not produce much in the way of functional SMN protein. The primary genetic feature, however, which determines the severity of SMA, seems to be the number of gene copies of *SMN2*, which is variable.[12] Studies have shown that a higher number of *SMN2* copies correlates with generally milder clinical phenotypes.[13]

Clinical Presentation

SMA is traditionally classified into 4 pediatric subtypes according to the age of onset and highest motor function achieved. Type 0 corresponds to a very severe form of antenatal-onset SMA. SMA type 1, also known as Werdnig-Hoffmann disease or infantile-onset SMA, is the most severe form of the disease (**Fig. 3**) and accounts for approximately 50% of patients.[14] Occasionally, there is a history of decreased intrauterine movements during pregnancy. Symptom onset is prior to 6 months of age

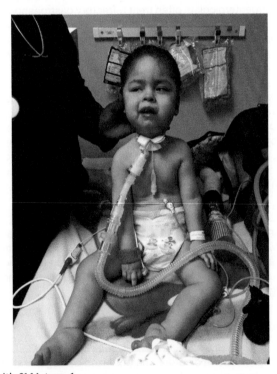

Fig. 3. Patient with SMA type 1.

and includes severe hypotonia, substantial muscle weakness with the inability to sit or stand, swallowing/feeding difficulties, and impaired breathing.

SMA type 2 develops between the 7 and 18 months of age.[15] The first sign is often a delay or regression of motor milestones. Patients suffer from significant hypotonia as well as muscle weakness with the lower extremities more affected than the upper extremities. Individuals with SMA type 2 typically can sit unsupported when placed but are unable walk independently (**Fig. 4**).[9]

SMA type 3, also known as Kugelberg-Welander disease, is typically diagnosed after 18 months of age. Individuals are initially able to walk but suffer from significant weakness leading to an increasing limitation of mobility as they grow. Most individuals eventually require the use of a wheelchair. Scoliosis can also develop.[9]

Physical Examination

The physical examination in any patient with SMA has common findings, including hypotonia and muscle weakness of varying degrees based on the type of SMA. Additional common findings include diminished to absent reflexes, the presence of tongue fasciculations (Video 1) and chest wall deformities.

Patients with SMA type 1 present very early in life with significant hypotonia and muscle wasting throughout. On occasion, arthrogryposis or scoliosis may be present at birth. On examination, these infants are often lying in a frog-legged position and demonstrate severe head lag and slip through with vertical suspension. Weakness can be profound with movements limited to distal muscle groups, such the hands and feet. Tongue fasciculations are almost always present in the course of the disease. Altered breathing patterns, including paradoxical breathing, are seen,

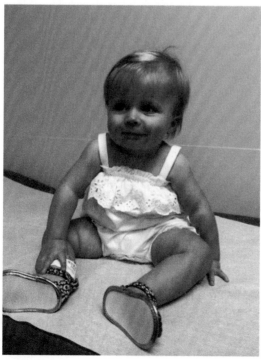

Fig. 4. Patient with SMA type 2.

sometimes even at presentation. Infants typically present with a weak cry and poor suck as well. A bell-shaped chest develops with time in direct proportion to respiratory weakness. Deep tendon reflexes are absent.

Patients with SMA type 2 also suffer from substantial hypotonia but less so when compared with infants with SMA type 1. Physical examination demonstrates head lag but with the ability of the patient to sit when placed. Patients may be able to lift arms partially against gravity but have little to no antigravity movements in the legs. Muscle atrophy is present throughout. Scoliosis as well as joint contractures develop with time. Tongue fasciculations may also be present as well as a fine tremor in fingers. Deep tendon reflexes are generally absent.

Patients with SMA type 3 present with varying degrees of hypotonia and muscle weakness. All patients achieve the ability to walk, however, even if for a limited amount of time. Muscle weakness is symmetric and affects the lower extremities more than upper extremities. Muscle atrophy is often present although on rare occasions, patients with SMA type 3 are noted to have increased muscle bulk of the calves. Patients demonstrate an abnormal gait with a Trendelenburg pattern. Tongue fasciculations are not typically present, although patients commonly have a tremor in outstretched hands. Deep tendon reflexes are diminished or absent.

Diagnostic Testing

If a provider is uncertain of the diagnosis at presentation, creatine kinase testing may be completed. Results are typically normal with the exception of patients with SMA type 3 who may have elevated CK of 2 times to 3 times normal. Most often, providers with a high clinical suspicion for SMA immediately recommend the *SMN* gene deletion test be performed. Testing is commonly completed by MLPA analysis. The test achieves up to 95% sensitivity and nearly 100% specificity.[16] A homozygous deletion of *SMN1* exon 7 (with or without deletion of exon 8) confirms the diagnosis.[9] If negative, providers may choose to perform additional testing including electromyography (EMG), nerve conduction studies, repetitive nerve stimulation and/or muscle biopsy because other, less common, variants of SMA (not discussed in this article) do exist. Should an EMG be performed on a patient with SMA, results demonstrate denervation with spontaneous activity of positive sharp waves, fibrillations, and occasional fasciculations as well as high amplitudes and long durations coupled with decreased recruitment in motor unit action potentials. Muscle biopsies reveal atrophic fibers with islands of group hypertrophy.[17]

Progression/Prognosis

Infants with SMA type 1 suffer from a rapid decline in respiratory and bulbar function. Without respiratory support, patients suffer from respiratory failure. Noninvasive ventilation combined with airway clearance techniques are generally supported. On occasion, however, ventilation assistance via tracheostomy and end-of-life discussions must be considered. Bulbar dysfunction resulting in dysphagia and/or gastroesophageal reflux must be managed either at diagnosis or shortly thereafter. A gastrostomy tube +/− Nissen fundoplication is often necessary to provide an infant with proper nutrition without posing the risk of aspiration. Infants typically suffer from constipation as well, which should be proactively managed to prevent impaction. Orthopedic concerns, including scoliosis and joint contractures, develop with time but are most often managed with supportive care given the risk of anesthesia. Infants with SMA may have evidence of autonomic dysfunction, including increased sweating and tachycardia. Cardiac disease, however, is not historically associated with SMA. Death from respiratory failure commonly occurs within the first 2 years of life.

Muscle weakness in patients with SMA type 2 is less progressive with time. Patients typically maintain the ability to sit, although they may only be able to sit with support as weakness evolves. Patients and their families may notice a decline in strength, particularly in the upper extremities. Changes of strength in the lower extremities are less obvious given that weakness is profound to begin with. Pulmonary disease is the major cause of morbidity and mortality in patients with SMA type 2. Patients with SMA type 2 suffer from restrictive lung disease that can lead to an impaired cough resulting in poor clearance of airway secretions, recurrent infections, and hypoventilation with sleep. Respiratory status can be directly related to the degree of scoliosis, which almost always occurs in patients with SMA type 2. Given the effects of scoliosis on pulmonary function, surgical correction is often warranted. Additional orthopedic concerns include joint contractures. Dysphagia occurs in a significant number of patients and swallow studies should be performed when indicated. Constipation is also a common concern. Life expectancy for patients with SMA type 2 is overall reduced although individuals can live into adulthood if pulmonary concerns are managed appropriately.

Patients with SMA type 3 often report a decline in strength with time. Many patients lose the ability to walk. Pulmonary disease should be regularly monitored but is not considered as prominent in patients with this form of disease. Dysphagia is less common as well. Scoliosis and joint contractures do occur in this population. Lifespan is typically normal.

Treatment Options

There are no approved treatments or a cure for patients with SMA. Patients are managed with supportive care. Care guidelines have been developed addressing the need for multidisciplinary care, including a neuromuscular specialist, pulmonologist, orthopedist, and gastroenterologist in efforts to provide quality care.[9]

Patients are typically seen by the neuromuscular team 2 to 3 times annually. In large academic centers, the team consists of a provider as well as physical, occupational, and speech therapy services and a registered dietician. At each visit, overall muscle strength and function are measured. Additionally, disease-associated concerns are addressed with particular attention to nutrition, gastrointestinal concerns, and orthopedic care. Referrals to specialists are placed as indicated.

In addition to the assessments discussed previously, patients with SMA should be regularly followed by a pulmonologist familiar with the management of neuromuscular disorders. When applicable, pulmonary function testing should be performed annually. Additionally, sleep studies are regularly recommended to screen for sleep-disordered breathing. Patients and families are educated regarding manually and mechanically assisted cough techniques and noninvasive ventilation, initially at night and then during the day as the disease progresses. As stated previously, assisted ventilation via tracheostomy may be considered as to prolong survival.

Research

Since 1995, scientists have known that a deficiency of functional SMN protein is the underlying cause of SMA. As discussed previously, 2 nearly identical genes carry the genetic instructions for the SMN protein: SMN1 and SMN2. Proteins made from the SMN1 gene are full-length and functional, and seem necessary for the survival and proper function of the motor neurons. By contrast, proteins made using instructions from the SMN2 gene are shorter and tend to be less stable. Researchers are seeking to take advantage of this unique redundancy through development of various strategies that restore sufficient levels of the needed full-length SMN protein from SMN2.[18] Specifically, gene therapy and the use of AONs are currently being investigated.

MYOTONIC DYSTROPHY
Overview

DM1 is a multisystem disease arising from mutant CTG expansion in the nontranslating region of the *DMPK* gene on chromosome 19q13.3. It is an autosomal dominant disorder with a worldwide prevalence of 1 in 8000.[19] Patients suffer from a wide array of symptoms given that the disease affects skeletal and smooth muscle as well as the eye, heart, endocrine system, and CNS. DM1 is characterized by anticipation, which is defined by increasing severity and earlier onset of the disease phenotype in successive generations related to the intergenerational expansion of the repeat size.[20]

There are 5 clinical phenotypes of DM1 that generally correlate with CTG repeat size; the higher the repeat, the more affected the individual. The 5 clinical phenotypes include premutation, mild adult myotonic dystrophy (DM), classical adult DM, childhood-onset DM, and congenital myotonic dystrophy (CDM).[19] For the purpose of this article, the discussion is limited to CDM and childhood-onset DM.

CDM is characterized by severe hypotonia and weakness at birth, often with respiratory insufficiency. The incidence of CDM is approximately 1 in 47,619 live births[21] and the mortality in the neonatal period may be as high as 30% to 40%.[20]

Childhood-onset DM is initially clinically apparent between ages 1 and 10 although diagnosis may occur later. DM1 in childhood most commonly affects muscle strength, cognition, respiratory system, CNS, and gastrointestinal system. Patients with childhood DM most often survive into adulthood.[20]

Clinical Presentation

Polyhydramnios, reduced fetal movements, and preterm delivery are associated with the gestational period of a neonate with CDM. Cases of small-for-gestational-age DM1 babies have also been reported. At birth, infants suffer from significant hypotonia and muscle weakness, a weak cry, and feeding, sucking and respiratory difficulties, often necessitating assisted ventilation, enteral feeds and admission to a neonatal ICU. Transmission occurs almost exclusively via the mother.[20]

Patients with childhood-onset DM1 are typically distinguished by a normal neonatal period. Brain involvement is a hallmark feature with learning difficulties as the main presenting symptom, resulting from various degrees of mental delay, psychopathologic manifestations, speech defects, hypersomnolence, and fatigue. The childhood form can be maternally or paternally inherited.[20]

Physical Examination

Physical examination of an infant with CDM demonstrates profound hypotonia and hyporeflexia in addition to severe muscle weakness. Infants may suffer from congenital contractures and/or arthrogryposis. Dysmorphic features include a tented mouth, ptosis, long neck and face, and temporal muscle atrophy.

In patients with childhood-onset DM, generalized hypotonia and arthrogryposis are the main clinical features, without respiratory distress. Bilateral isolated clubfeet could be the first isolated sign of the disease. Muscle weakness of varying degrees is also a common feature. Muscle weakness is more pronounced distally in patients with DM1. Facial weakness, including a high narrow palate, ptosis, and/or temporal muscle atrophy, is also often present (**Fig. 5**). In patients older than 5 years of age, grip myotonia and/or percussion myotonia may be present.

Diagnostic Testing

Serum CK testing is typically normal to minimally elevated. EMG is of little assistance in neonates given that myotonic discharges are not present prior to 5 or 6 years of age

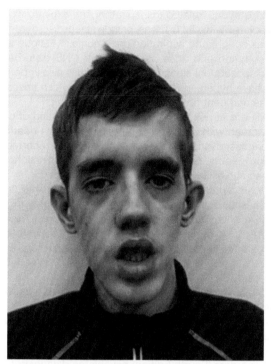

Fig. 5. Patient with DM1 demonstrating typical myopathic facies.

but may be a useful diagnostic tool in older patients with suspicion for childhood-onset DM1 or in parents who may have transmitted the disease. Pathology from a muscle biopsy may demonstrate myopathic features, including centralized nuclei. Ultimately, a diagnosis of DM1 is made by molecular techniques that can demonstrate the CTG expansion in *DMPK*.

Neuroimaging studies are also important in patients with DM1 and may demonstrate ventricular dilatation, diffuse cerebral atrophy, wide Virchow-Robin spaces, and subcortical white matter abnormalities.[20]

Progression/Prognosis

Severe CDM demonstrates a unique biphasic course, whereby neonatal symptoms improve or stabilize in surviving neonates, before adult-type symptoms present in later life.[22] Therefore, surviving CDM neonates and childhood-onset DM1 patients share common but varying degrees of clinical manifestations with time.

As stated previously, muscle weakness in DM1 is typically distal but may also include proximal muscle groups, the latter indicating a poorer prognosis.[23] The natural history of muscle weakness in patients with CDM and childhood-onset DM is variable. Most commonly, strength is often stable prior to adolescence with gradual deterioration or, rarely, rapid increased weakness is present in young adults.[24] Clinical signs of myotonia develop after 5 years of age, including grip myotonia and percussion myotonia. Bulbar weakness is frequently present, producing swallowing and speech/language difficulties. Complications of widespread muscle weakness can also lead to orthopedic abnormalities, including joint contractures and scoliosis.

Respiratory manifestations, related to inspiratory and expiratory muscle weakness, are commonly associated with DM1. These include sleep-disordered breathing, recurrent infections, weak cough, and aspiration pneumonia.[24] Fatigue and daytime somnolence are also common and arise as a result of CNS disturbances resulting in hypoventilation and subsequent sleep fragmentation. It is also important to appreciate that DM1 patients have hypersensitivity to anesthesia, which arises from respiratory muscle compromise and central dysregulation of breathing.[25]

Patients with DM1 are at risk for cardiac disease consisting of conduction disturbances that may worsen with time and can result in sudden death. In pediatric patients, disabling cardiac dysfunction or arrhythmias are reported to be silent or discrete. Conduction defects, however, can be diagnosed in childhood, thus necessitating proper cardiac surveillance including Holter monitors.[26]

Gastrointestinal complaints are present in almost all patients with DM1. Factors include reduced peristalsis and secondary bacterial overgrowth. Studies suggest that 40% of children and young adults regularly experience fecal incontinence[27] and up to one-third report constipation and/or irregular bowel habits.[28] Dysphagia and gastroesophageal reflux may be present as a consequence of bulbar weakness (described previously). Lastly, nausea, vomiting and early satiety can be attributed to delayed gastric emptying.

Essentially all pediatric patients with DM1 suffer from cognitive deficits and/or impaired psychosocial function. CDM patients are more severely affected and full-scale IQ ranges from 40 to 80, with a mean below 70.[29] Childhood-onset patients have a wider range of IQs, from 42 to 114, and a mean of approximately 70 to 80.[30] Approximately half of children with DM1 have at least 1 *Diagnostic and Statistical Manual of Mental Disorders* (Fourth Edition) psychiatric diagnosis.[31] Internalizing disorders, including phobias, depression, and anxiety, as well as attention-deficit/hyperactivity disorders are common. Additionally, autistic spectrum disorders have been reported in up to 49% of patients.[32]

Endocrine abnormalities are also commonly found in patients with DM1, although less in the pediatric population compared with adults. Testicular atrophy and infertility are common in CDM male patients. Female patients with severe CDM may experience very irregular periods and prolonged episodes of amenorrhea. Hypothyroidism, hypogonadism, growth hormone imbalance, and androgen insensitivity have been observed but are rare.[33] Diabetes mellitus may occur as well.

Other key features that are important to recognize in patients with DM1 include the risk of cataracts. Lens pathology may be evident in 41% of patients and may be predictive of future cataract development.[34]

Treatment Options

Treatment of DM1 is limited to supportive care with an overall goal to manage patients' symptoms and comorbidities, optimize function of the patient, and assist in health surveillance. Management should include a multidisciplinary care team of health care professionals, including multiple medical specialties; physical, occupational, and speech therapists; registered dieticians; and social workers.

Neuromuscular specialists or pediatric neurologists commonly follow patients with CDM or childhood-onset DM. Patients require ongoing evaluations by clinicians as well as physical and occupational therapists to assess and maximize function. A home exercise program, including stretching, orthoses, and assistive devices, may be indicated.

Multiple medications have undergone research to determine if they are helpful in decreasing symptoms of myotonia, which may include decreased dexterity, gait instability, difficulty with speech/swallowing, and muscle pain. An article published in 2010 concluded that mexiletine, at dosages of 150 mg and 200 mg 3 times daily, was effective, safe, and well-tolerated over 7 weeks as an antimyotonia treatment in DM1.[35] The study was limited, however, to adult patients and similar studies in the pediatric population are nonexistent.

Regular respiratory and cardiac surveillance is important children with DM1. Similarly to the other diagnoses discussed previously, patients should undergo regular pulmonary function testing. Airway clearance techniques are beneficial in management of a weak cough. Polysomnograms are indicated for daytime fatigue or sleep concerns. Noninvasive ventilation may improve quality of life when there is hypoventilation or apnea. Bilevel positive airway pressure (BiPAP) use is first line. Routine electrocardiography, echocardiogram, and Holter monitoring should be routinely performed to assess for arrhythmias. Cardiac interventions, such as a pacemaker or implanted defibrillator, are indicated when needed.

Patients may also require referrals to orthopedics and gastroenterology if indicated. Neuropsychological testing is helpful given cognitive and psychological concerns. Lastly, genetic counseling can assist with family planning discussions.

Research

Research opportunities for patients with myotonic dystrophy include multiple molecular therapeutic approaches, which target the mutant, expanded RNA. AONs complementary to target mutations are synthesized, in the hope that the target mutant sequence is silenced. Additionally, AONs have been used in an attempt to degrade the RNA expansions and the mutant *DMPK* allele through enzymatic actions. Studies looking specifically at reducing muscle weakness by introducing anabolic stimuli have also been performed. Agents studied include testosterone, creatine, dehydroepiandrosterone, and recombinant insulinlike growth factor. Studies have yet to show improvements, however, in muscle function in patients.

SUMMARY

Pediatric patients often present to a primary care provider with concerns for developmental delay, hypotonia, and/or muscle weakness. It is important for pediatric providers to effectively recognize neuromuscular diseases as a potential cause for symptoms. Most neuromuscular diseases have been historically viewed as untreatable. Recent medical advances, however, in pulmonary and cardiac care have significantly improved the life span for many disorders. Additionally, new potential therapeutics have promising results, making early diagnosis imperative.

SUPPLEMENTARY DATA

Supplementary data related to this article can be found online at http://dx.doi.org/10.1016/j.cpha.2016.05.002.

REFERENCES

1. Emery AE. Population frequencies of inherited neuromuscular diseases – a world survey. Neuromuscul Disord 1991;1:19–29.
2. Stark AE. Determinants of the incidence of Duchenne muscular dystrophy. Ann Transl Med 2015;3(19):287.
3. Aartsma-Rus A, Ginjaar IB, Bushby K. The importance of genetic diagnosis for Duchenne muscular dystrophy. J Med Genet 2016;53(3):145–51.

4. MdAdam L. Cognitive and neurobehavioral profile in boys with Duchenne muscular dystrophy. J Child Neurol 2015;30(11):1472–82.
5. Bushby KM, Goodship JA, Nicholson LV, et al. Variability in clinical, genetic and protein abnormalities in manifesting carriers of Duchenne and Becker muscular dystrophy. Neuromuscul Disord 1993;3:57–64.
6. Pestronk A. Duchenne muscular dystrophy. Washington University Neuromuscular Center. Available at: http://neuromuscular.wustl.edu/. Accessed February 5, 2016.
7. Bushby K, Finkel R, Birnkrant DJ, et al. Diagnosis and management of Duchenne muscular dystrophy, part 1: diagnosis, and pharmacological and psychosocial management. Lancet Neurol 2010;9:77–93.
8. Bushby K, Finkel R, Birnkrant DJ, et al. Diagnosis and management of Duchenne muscular dystrophy, part 2: Implementation of multidisciplinary care. Lancet Neurol 2010;9:177–89.
9. Wang CH, Finkel RS, Bertini ES, et al. Consensus statement for standard of care in spinal muscular atrophy. J Child Neurol 2007;8:1027–49.
10. Ogino S, Leonard DG, Rennert H, et al. Genetic risk assessment in carrier testing for spinal muscular atrophy. Am J Med Genet 2002;110:301–7.
11. Nicole S, Diaz CC, Frugier T, et al. Spinal muscular atrophy: recent advances and future prospects. Muscle Nerve 2002;26:4–13.
12. Prior T. Perspectives and diagnostic considerations in spinal muscular atrophy. Genet Med 2010;12:145–52.
13. Campbell L, Potter A, Ignatius J, et al. Genetic variation and gene conversion in spinal muscular atrophy: implications for disease process and clinical phenotype. Am J Hum Genet 1997;61:40–50.
14. Markowitz JA, Tinkle MG, Fishbeck KH. Spinal muscular atrophy in the neonate. J Obstet Gynecol Neonatal Nurs 2004;33:12–20.
15. Lunn MR, Wang CH. Spinal muscular atrophy. Lancet 2008;371:2120–33.
16. Rodrigues NR, Owen N, Talbot K, et al. Deletions in the survival motor neuron gene on 5q13 in autosomal recessive spinal muscular atrophy. Hum Mol Genet 1995;4:631–4.
17. Buchthal F, Olsen PZ. Electromyography and muscle biopsy in infantile spinal muscular atrophy. Brain 1970;93:15–30.
18. Muscular Dystrophy Association. Spinal muscular atrophy: research. 2016. Available at: https://www.mda.org/disease/spinal-muscular-atrophy/research. Accessed February 19, 2016.
19. Ho G, Cardamone M, Farrar M. Congenital and childhood myotonic dystrophy: current aspects of disease and future directions. World J Clin Pediatr 2015; 4(4):66–80.
20. Echenne B, Bassez G. Congenital and infantile myotonic dystrophy. Handb Clin Neurol 2013;113:1387–93.
21. Campbell C, Levin S, Siu VM, et al. Congenital myotonic dystrophy: Canadian population-based surveillance study. J Pediatr 2013;163:120–5.
22. Hageman AT, Gabreëls FJ, Liem KD, et al. Congenital myotonic dystrophy; a report on thirteen cases and a review of the literature. J Neurol Sci 1993;115: 95–101.
23. Mathieu J, Allard P, Potvin L, et al. A 10-year study of mortality in a cohort of patients with myotonic dystrophy. Neurology 1999;52:1658–62.
24. Echenne B, Rideau A, Roubertie A, et al. Myotonic dystrophy type I in childhood long-term evolution in patients surviving the neonatal period. Eur J Paediatr Neurol 2008;12:210–23.

25. Veyckemans F, Scholtes JL. Myotonic dystrophies type 1 and 2: anesthetic care. Paediatr Anaesth 2013;23:794–803.
26. Bassez G, Lazarus A, Desguerre I, et al. Severe cardiac arrhythmias in young patients with myotonic dystrophy type 1. Neurology 2004;63:1939–41.
27. Kerr TP, Robb SA, Clayden GS. Lower gastrointestinal tract disturbance in congenital myotonic dystrophy. Eur J Pediatr 2002;161:468–9.
28. Reardon W, Newcombe R, Fenton I, et al. The natural history of congenital myotonic dystrophy: mortality and long term clinical aspects. Arch Dis Child 1993;68: 177–81.
29. Harper PS. Myotonic dystrophy. 3rd edition. London: W.B. Saunders; 2001.
30. Angeard N, Gargiulo M, Jacquette A, et al. Cognitive profile in childhood myotonic dystrophy type 1: is there a global impairment? Neuromuscul Disord 2007;17: 451–8.
31. Douniol M, Jacquette A, Cohen D, et al. Psychiatric and cognitive phenotype of childhood myotonic dystrophy type 1. Dev Med Child Neurol 2012;54:905–11.
32. Ekström AB, Hakenäs-Plate L, Samuelsson L, et al. Autism spectrum conditions in myotonic dystrophy type 1: a study on 57 individuals with congenital and childhood forms. Am J Med Genet B Neuropsychiatr Genet 2008;147B:918–26.
33. O'Brien TA, Harper PS. Course, prognosis and complications of childhood-onset myotonic dystrophy. Dev Med Child Neurol 1984;26:62–7.
34. Ekström AB, Tulinius M, Sjöström A, et al. Visual function in congenital and childhood myotonic dystrophy type 1. Ophthalmology 2010;117:976–82.
35. Logigian EL, Martens WB, Moxley RT, et al. Mexiletine is an effective antimyotonia treatment in myotonic dystrophy type 1. Neurology 2010;74:1441–8.

Evaluation of Pediatric Toe Walking

Courtney Bishop, MPAS, PA-C

KEYWORDS

- Toe walking • Idiopathic toe walking • Cerebral palsy • Muscular dystrophies

KEY POINTS

- Persistent toe walking in a child older than 2 years warrants evaluation and investigation by a medical provider.
- Idiopathic toe walking is a diagnosis of exclusion and is the most common cause of pediatric toe walking.
- A thorough patient history and physical examination is required to determine the cause of the toe walking or to diagnose idiopathic toe walking.
- Toe walking from an identified neurologic or neurogenic cause should be sent to a specialist for further evaluation and management.
- Although statistically most children will grow out of idiopathic toe walking, families may have significant concerns, and conservative or surgical treatment may be beneficial.

INTRODUCTION

Toe walking, or lack of heel contact with the floor during the initial stance phase of the gait cycle, or absence of complete foot contact during the gait cycle, is a common concern for parents of young children and is often brought to the attention of medical providers.[1,2] Although bilateral toe walking is often considered normal for toddlers as they establish their gait, consistent toe walking in a child older than 2 to 3 years or asymmetric toe walking warrants further evaluation by a medical provider.[3] There are multiple potential causes of toe walking that must be considered by the provider and include, but are not limited to, idiopathic toe walking (ITW), cerebral palsy (CP), muscular dystrophies, leg length discrepancy, or trauma (**Box 1**).

IDIOPATHIC TOE WALKING

Toe walking in otherwise healthy children and apparent normal development was first described in 1967 by Hall and colleagues.[4] ITW is a diagnosis of exclusion and is often defined as continued and consistent equinus gait after 3 years of age in the absence of

Disclosure: None.
Department of Orthopaedics, Nationwide Children's Hospital, 700 Children's Ave., Suite T2E-A2700, Columbus, OH 43205, USA
E-mail address: Courtney.bishop@nationwidechildrens.org

Physician Assist Clin 1 (2016) 599–613
http://dx.doi.org/10.1016/j.cpha.2016.05.006   **physicianassistant.theclinics.com**

Box 1
Toe walking differentials

- Idiopathic toe walking
  - Habitual
  - Anatomic
- Neurologic
  - Central nervous system
    - CP
    - Spinal cord lesion
  - Muscular dystrophy
    - Duchenne
    - Becker
- LLD
  - Premature physeal closure
    - Injury
    - Infection
  - Developmental dysplasia of the hip
  - Congenital
    - Hemihypertrophy
    - Congenital femoral deficiency
    - Fibular hemimelia

Associated diagnostic differentials

- Autism spectrum disorder
- Developmental delay
  - Gross motor
  - Speech
  - Learning

---

a known medical condition.[1,2,4–7] Although originally considered solely caused by a contracture or shortening of the Achilles tendon,[4] it has since been found that many children who toe walk do not have a concomitant Achilles contracture.[1,5] There are currently multiple theories as to the pathophysiology of ITW; however, there is no true known cause. In 1978, Montgomery and Gauger[8] suggested that ITW might be a result of children in developed nations having a defect in sensory processing because of their lack of time spent barefoot. Williams and colleagues[9] postulated that ITW occurs because of a defect in sensory processing either because of a vestibular disorder or an abnormal sensitivity to touch. Additionally, ITW is suggested to have a myopathic process owing to increased proportions of type 1 muscle fibers from gastrocnemius muscle biopsies compared with the normal findings of primarily type 2 muscle fibers in the gastrocnemius in non–toe walkers.[10]

There are limited data on the incidence of toe walking in the pediatric population; however, multiple studies have estimated its prevalence. Historically, ITW is estimated to occur anywhere between 7% and 24% of the childhood population.[11,12] A study by Engelbert and colleagues[11] in 2011 found a prevalence of ITW with a cross-sectional study in 12% of the childhood population in the Netherlands. In 2012, Engstrom and Tedroff[13] approximated the prevalence of children in Sweden with a reported history of toe walking before 5.5 years of age to be 4.87%, with only 2.09% of 5.5 year olds being active toe walkers. The findings of Engstrom and Tedroff[13] suggested that in the absence of a comorbidity, most children would establish a normal gait pattern by 5.5 years of age.[13]

For ITW to be diagnosed, multiple anatomic, neurogenic, and neuromuscular causes must first be ruled out. Providers must be able to effectively evaluate the child for potential differential diagnoses to determine if a patient is an idiopathic toe walker and if treatment or referral is required.

NONIDIOPATHIC CAUSES OF TOE WALKING

Toe walking can be caused by a variety of factors, both anatomic and physiologic. The Achilles tendon is formed from the gastrocnemius and soleus muscles and inserts on the posterior calcaneus. The convergence of the gastrocnemius and soleus muscles with the Achilles tendon is known anatomically as the triceps surae muscle-tendon complex.[6] Increased plantar flexion of the foot secondary to overactivity of the triceps surae complex is known as an equinus deformity of the foot and can be either flexible or fixed. Toe walkers may have an equinus deformity causing their toe-toe gait because of their inability to dorsiflex the foot appropriately. Contractures of the knee or hip joints may also cause toe walking because of a shortening of the leg length compared with the contralateral, therefore, forcing the child to walk on his or her toes with a crouched gait to equal the length of the contralateral leg.

Cerebral Palsy

CP is a neuromuscular disorder caused by a fixed and nonprogressive brain lesion that causes motor impairment but is found without injury or biomechanical abnormality to the spinal cord or muscles.[14] Brain injury that results in CP can occur at any time before age 5, including in the prenatal or perinatal periods. Spastic diplegic CP is the most common cause of toe walking other than ITW.[15] CP generally causes increased spasticity and muscle tone as well as joint contractures in the affected lower extremity. Other central nervous system and neuromuscular disorders that can cause or present with toe walking include spinal cord abnormalities such as tumors, tethered cord, syringomeyelia, or spina bifida, as well as Charcot-Marie-Tooth neuropathy or dystonias.[16]

Muscular Dystrophies

Both Duchenne and Becker muscular dystrophies may cause children to walk on their toes to compensate for weakness of the knee extensors, which, in turn, can cause progressive contractures of the Achilles.[16] Other signs and symptoms that may be suggestive of muscular dystrophies are large calf muscles, complaints of muscle pains or stiffness, trouble running and jumping, a waddling gait, and difficulty getting up from a lying or seated position.[17] Duchenne and Becker muscular dystrophies can present with similar symptoms; however, symptoms of Duchenne muscular dystrophy present at an earlier age (mostly between 2 and 3 years of age), are more severe, and progresses more rapidly than Becker muscular dystrophy.[17] Symptoms of Becker muscular dystrophy often begin appearing when the patient is a teenager.

Leg Length Discrepancy

A child may also toe walk because of a difference in the lengths of his or her legs. This condition can be caused by a variety of factors, both true and apparent. True limb length discrepancy (LLD) of the legs can be secondary to either premature arrest of a physis or multiple physes or caused by a congenital disorder of the leg causing asymmetric growth. Premature physeal arrest is often caused by trauma, which can be secondary to infection or injury, including septic joint, osteomyelitis, traumas, juvenile arthritis, compartment syndrome, neurofibromatosis, or Ollier's disease.

Congenital disorders such as hemihypertrophy, congenital femoral deficiency, or fibular hemimelia may also cause an LLD, triggering the child to toe walk to accommodate for their limb length difference.

An additionally important differential in the growing child to evaluate for possible causes of LLD is developmental dysplasia of the hip (DDH). Congenital dislocation of the hip occurs at birth when the acetabulum of the hip and the femur are both underdeveloped. If the dislocation is not corrected within the first few weeks of life, the hip joint cannot develop appropriately. Although screening for DDH has increased in recent years, DDH can be first noticed by parents when children are around 1 year of age and begin ambulating, with it appearing as if the child is limping or toe walking.[18]

Developmental Delay

Multiple studies found that there is an increased prevalence of toe walking in individuals with developmental, language, and learning delays.[1,19,20] Additionally, there is an increased prevalence of persistent toe walking in children with autism spectrum disorder than in the overall population, with incidence approximately 20%.[21] Children with autism spectrum disorder can also present with other physical or repetitive stereotypes including lack of eye contact, eye gazing, finger flicking, and persistent sniffing or licking. Autism is usually reliably diagnosed in children by age 3 years, and medical providers should consider it a potential concomitant diagnosis in a child with persistent toe walking.[22]

PATIENT EXAMINATION
History

A complete medical history of the child should be obtained that includes prenatal and birth histories, developmental milestones, and any known history of illnesses or injuries. Significant pre- and perinatal historical information includes length of pregnancy, any infections or medical issues with mother during the pregnancy, whether the child was a product of a single or multiple births, length of labor, method of patient delivery, infant position at birth, and birth weight. Postnatal complications or whether there was a required neonatal intensive care stay may also be significant. CP is more common in multiple births, premature children, children with a low birth weight, and those that sustained perinatal brain injuries including stroke, hemorrhage, or asphyxia. A recent retrospective study by Baber and colleagues[23] in Australia found that children with ITW have higher rates of pre- and postnatal complications than the general population, suggesting that there could be a neurologic cause secondary to a mild neurologic insult.

Children follow a predictable course of developmental milestones of gross motor control with a culmination in functional independent ambulation and mobility. Ages for each milestone are expected for the 50th percentile of age, with accepted and expected deviation for individuals. To appropriately assess a pediatric patient to determine the nature of toe walking, the provider must be aware of the gross motor milestones that patients should be meeting at any given age.

Ambulatory gross motor milestones then begin with cruising and walking with 2 hands held at 10 months, taking independent steps at 12 months, and walking without arms out for balance at approximately 14 months.[24] At approximately 12 months of age, children may begin to demonstrate hand dominance. Hand dominance before 1 year of age can be suggestive of hemiplegic CP.[20] By 20 months, children often run well and can walk up and down stairs with a hand held.[25] An estimated 95% of children begin independent ambulation between 10 and 17 months of age. A toddler's gait is noted to lack a consistent rhythm and symmetry, with a broad base. Toe walking can be a normal gait pattern in children younger than 3 years until their gait is fully established. At 3 years, children should have developed a synchronous gait and a heel-to-toe gait.[24] A fully established and adult-type gait pattern is often established by 6 to 7 years of age.[20,24]

Especially in children being evaluated for a concern of toe walking, the provider should investigate the age at which the child began walking independently and if the child had an established gait before the onset of toe walking. Toe walking may present at any stage during the development of gait, including with prewalking skills, the start of prewalking, or within 6 months of independent walking, and is considered persistent once it lasts longer than 3 months after the onset of independent ambulation.[6,21,25] The family should be questioned regarding the proportion of time the child spends toe walking, if the child can walk flat footed when prompted, and the nature of the toe walking.

If a child's toe walking began after a previously established gait, if there are parental concerns of a limp, or if the child is complaining of pain, suspicions must be raised for a potential injury or trauma to the foot. Differential diagnoses should include fractures to the affected lower extremity or the presence of a foreign body in the foot. Studies note that pain in the foot or leg can be a concern in patients who may have ITW.[3,25,26]

Toe walking in a child who previously had an established gait without complaints of pain or limp is highly concerning of a progressive neuromuscular disorder including muscular dystrophies, Charcot-Marie-Tooth neuropathy, spinal cord lesions, or tethered cord.[3,15,16]

Family reports that the child has toe walked since the initiation of their gait is more suggestive of ITW, an LLD, or a static neuromuscular condition, such as CP.[25] Children with ITW are more likely to intermittently toe walk, stand plantigrade, and be able to demonstrate a heel-toe gait.[25]

Bilateral toe walking is more consistent with a diagnosis of ITW, muscular dystrophies, or autism. If the child has only walked on their toes unilaterally, concern for LLD, DDH, dystonia, or hemiplegic CP is raised.

The provider should elicit from parents if there is any family history of toe walking. In children with ITW, there is often a positive family history of toe walking, as evidenced in multiple cross-sectional and case studies.[4–6,12,26,27] Additionally, there is often a positive family history in children with DDH and genetic conditions such as congenital muscular dystrophies, skeletal dysplasias, and sickle cell disorders, all of which could be potential causes of toe walking.

Family should be asked if the child has been experiencing any additional symptoms. These symptoms could include neurologic symptoms such as changes in bowel or bladder control or complaints of numbness or tingling in either or both lower extremities. Changes in weight, appetite, or sleeping habits and recent fevers, chills, or nighttime sweats should also be questioned to evaluate for possible symptoms of malignancy.

Physical Examination

To fully evaluate a child that toe walks or to determine if the child meets the diagnosis of exclusion of ITW, a thorough musculoskeletal and neurologic examination must be performed. The child should be barefoot, dressed in only shorts or gown, with their knees and feet exposed.

The patient should stand straight, with their feet flat on the ground when possible and their back to the provider to assess for pelvic height. The patient should not have one knee hyperflexed compared with the other. This is a quick assessment for gross LLD and pelvic asymmetry. True assessment of an LLD is determined clinically with the patient standing or lying down, by measuring the length of the leg from the anterior superior iliac spine to the medial malleolus of the ankle with a tape measure.[28] An alternative method for determining difference in leg length is having the child stand and placing premeasured blocks under the shorter leg until the pelvis is level, therefore determining the LLD.

The Trendelenburg test is performed by having the child (if developmentally able) stand first on one leg and then the other. When a child stands on a leg with gluteal weakness, the child's hip will tilt toward the unaffected leg and can be seen unilaterally or bilaterally in DDH or with muscular dystrophies.[29]

The spine should be inspected for cutaneous abnormalities including sacral dimples, hair tufts, or midline pigmented or vascular lesions, which may be suggestive of an underlying spinal cord disorder.

The Gower's sign can be evaluated by having the child sit on the floor and asking them to stand. A positive Gower's sign is present when a child uses their hands to walk up their lower extremities to a standing position and cannot do so otherwise because of proximal muscle weakness. If a child exhibits a positive Gower's sign, it is suggestive of a congenital muscular dystrophy.[16,17]

The child should then lie in a supine position on an examination table. The Galeazzi test is performed by first flexing the hip and knees up so the child's feet are flat on the table, and placing their feet side-to-side with their heels level and touching their buttocks. The height of their knees should be equal—any discrepancy in the height of the knees is suggestive of an LLD.

Examination of the child's hips begins with abducting the hips, with the hips and knees extended, with the child in a supine position (**Fig. 1**). Normal abduction of the hips with legs extended is 45°.[29] Abduction of the hips should be symmetric. Asymmetric abduction of the hips is suggestive of either unilateral DDH or contracture of the abductors of the hip, which is common in children with hemiplegic CP. Additionally, internal and external rotation of the hips, with the child either supine or prone, should be symmetric. Passively flexing the patient's hip and knee to the chest and observing the contralateral leg for spontaneous passive flexion is the Thomas test and, when positive, indicates a hip flexion contracture. If a child has a significant hip flexion contracture, they may compensate for the contracture by altering their gait, flexing their knee, and ambulating on their toes on the affected side.

Evaluation of hamstring tightness is performed with the child in a supine position, passively flexing the hip to a 90° angle while holding the child's foot in one hand and the child's contralateral thigh with the other (**Fig. 2**). The leg is then gently extended until there is a catch from hamstring tightness. This angle is known as *the anterior popliteal angle* and is measured between the thigh and the shin. Expected anterior popliteal angles in children 1 to 3 years of age is 0° to 15° and for older children may range from 0° to 50°. In any child, an anterior popliteal angle greater than 50° shows hamstring tightness.[30] Hamstring tightness or contractures can cause a child to walk with a crouched gait and may eventually lead to a fixed knee flexion contracture.

Normal range of motion of the ankle is 40° of plantar flexion to 20° of dorsiflexion.[6] To determine if there is a contracture or tightness of the triceps surae, it is best to have the patient in a supine position. The hip and knee should be kept in extended positions, and the foot should first be inverted with the provider's hand to lock the subtalar joint and, therefore, prevent dorsiflexion of the midfoot. Dorsiflexion of the ankle is then tested, and the angle that is measured is formed from the anterior shaft of the

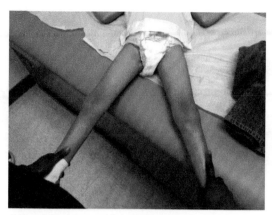

Fig. 1. Abduction of hips with hips and knees extended.

tibia and the lateral border of the foot (**Fig. 3**). Normal ankle dorsiflexion with the knee extended is 10° to 15° greater than neutral. If the ankle cannot be dorsiflexed to greater than 10° greater than neutral, it is suggestive of an Achilles contracture. If the patient does show a decreased measurement less than normal, the examination should then be repeated with the hip and knee in flexion to determine the involvement of the gastrocnemius muscle alone versus the triceps surae complex. Because the gastrocnemius crosses the knee joint but the soleus does not, a significant difference in the measurements is indicative that the gastrocnemius is the tight component of the triceps surae complex, and the patient has a gastrocnemius contracture, not an Achilles contracture. This examination technique is known as *the Silfverskiold test*. It is generally accepted that for a normal heel strike in an individual's gait, ankle dorsiflexion must at least be 10° greater than neutral.

The foot should then be evaluated for any deformities and, if present, whether they are fixed or flexible. Children with ITW and tight Achilles may have midtarsal pronation with weight bearing.[31] A cavus deformity of the foot is suggestive of a neurologic disorder.[16] Hindfoot varus in a toe walker is often caused by the tibialis posterior or tibialis

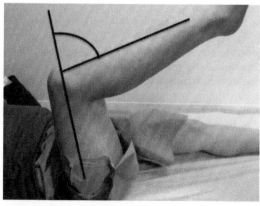

Fig. 2. Measurement of anterior popliteal angle.

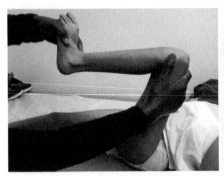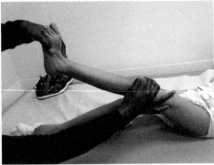

Fig. 3. Silfverskiold test to evaluate for gastrocnemius tightness.

anterior tendons being overactive secondary to spasticity and, again, may be suggestive of a neurologic disorder.

While examining the child's lower extremities, the overall quality and tone of the musculature should be noted. Bilateral hypertrophy of the calves is suggestive of a muscular dystrophy. Atrophy of the muscles may be suggestive of a neuromuscular disorder, previous trauma or infection, or congenital hemimelia. Increased tone is indicates an upper motor neuron injury or lesion such as CP or spinal cord injury.[32] Spasticity is velocity dependent, and is tested for by quickly passively moving the joint through its range of motion. If the muscles are spastic, they will "catch" with rapid movement but have greater range of motion with slow and steady movement. Hypotonia may also be present and is suggestive of a lower motor neuron or cerebellar lesion.

A complete neurologic examination of the entire body should be performed with evaluation of motor and sensory function of all extremities. Reflexes to be examined include triceps, biceps, patellar, and Achilles deep tendon reflexes; abdominal reflexes in all 4 quadrants; and the Babinski reflex. Deep tendon reflexes should be symmetric, and any evidence of hyperreflexia or hyporeflexia could be suggestive of central nervous system damage or peripheral neuropathy, respectively. Asymmetric abdominal reflexes may be suggestive of an intraspinal abnormality.[29] Clonus should also be examined for in the bilateral lower extremities by quickly dorsiflexing the ankle with the hip and knee flexed. The presence of clonus is highly suggestive of an underlying neurologic disorder.

One of the most important aspects of the physical examination in a child with concern of toe walking is evaluation of their gait. Especially in the pediatric population, it is often advantageous to observe the patient walk while they are unaware their gait is being evaluated. Otherwise, the child may develop anxiety and refuse to ambulate, may walk with a heel-toe gait because they know they are supposed to, or run or skip instead of demonstrating their standard gait. Therefore, attempting to observe the child as they walk into the examination room or examining their gait while they interact with family in the examination room, without drawing attention to their gait, may prove beneficial.

The gait cycle is divided into 2 main components: the stance phase and the swing phase (Fig. 4). The stance phase is the time during which the foot makes contact with the ground and the swing phase is the time during which the foot advances forward in the air. The stance phase is divided into 3 different components, also known as the 3 rockers. The first stage is initial contact, or double limb support, which begins with the heel strike and the first rocker with the ankle in plantar flexion.[6,29] The second stage is single limb stance, in which the foot is flat on the ground, with the ankle dorsiflexing in relation to the tibia in the second rocker. Finally, with pre-swing or toe-off, the toes leave the ground as the ankle plantar flexes.[6,29] Individuals who toe walk lack the initial heel strike portion of the gait, which loads the foot, and lack the transfer of body weight through the foot, instead remaining in equinus throughout the stance phase.[26,32]

Evaluation of the child's gait should include observation of the hips, legs, and knees as well as the ankles and feet. The examiner should be evaluating for other possible conditions while assessing the nature of the child's toe walking. A Trendelenburg gait with unequal swaying laterally is caused by gluteal weakness and is suggestive of a hip condition or muscular dystrophy.[16,29] Asymmetric movement of the knees, locked knees, or knees that hyperextend with gait may be suggestive of hemiplegic CP, a fixed knee contracture, or a tight Achilles, respectively.[32] In a child who can heel-toe walk when prompted, the patient may be noted to pronate or externally rotate the affected foot, with or without foot abduction, to compensate for an equinus contracture.[32] A midfoot break may occur during the gait cycle in older children with a history of toe walking, as a compensatory mechanism, and is more frequently seen when there is a neuromuscular disorder than in children with ITW.[3]

DIAGNOSTIC TESTING

If imaging or further testing is indicated based on physical examination, it is often beneficial to start with plain radiographs. Standing, full-length, anteroposterior radiographs of the bilateral lower extremities with a magnetic marker are best to measure a child's lower limb lengths and are generally considered more accurate than clinical measurements.[28] Additionally, with these radiographs, any premature physeal closure could be seen in the lower extremities. Anteroposterior films of the pelvis can show any subluxation or dislocation of the hip that would suggest developmental hip dysplasia. If a patient did have an acute onset of toe walking after having previously

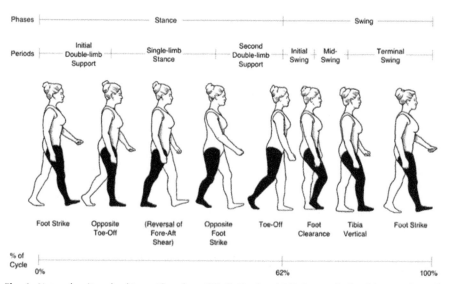

Fig. 4. Normal gait cycle. (*From* Chambers HG, Sutherland DH. A practical guide to gait analysis. J Am Acad Orthop Surg 2002;10:229; with permission.)

established a heel-toe gait, plain radiographs of the foot and ankle may be beneficial to evaluate for foreign bodies or potential fracture. In young children, when fracture is suspected, it is important to remember that occult fractures may not be visible on initial radiographs because of the highly cartilaginous make up of their bones; repeat radiographs in 10 to 14 days may show periosteal reaction, supporting a healing fracture or injury.

If there is concern for a neurologic or neuromuscular cause of the toe walking, MRI of the brain or spine, or both, is the most appropriate test to evaluate for any lesions or abnormalities, and the child should be referred to a pediatric neurologist or neurosurgeon.

Electromyography (EMG) gait studies can be performed to further evaluate gait, whether for gaining further information regarding the patient's gait or for surgical planning by an orthopedic surgeon. In children with ITW or CP, EMG gait studies find abnormalities in the gastrocnemius and anterior tibialis that persist even with the child attempting to walk with a heel-toe gait pattern.[33,34] EMG gait studies, however, are not consistently reliable in differentiating between a diagnosis of ITW and CP and are, therefore, not often deemed necessary in determining the cause of a child's toe walking.[34,35]

In patients for whom muscular dystrophy is a potential differential diagnosis, whether because of family history, a positive Gower's sign, or progressive weakness, creatine kinase levels are a first-line test to rule out a muscular dystrophy. A normal creatine kinase level indicates that the patient does not have a muscular dystrophy diagnosis. However, when there is a significant concern for a muscular dystrophy, a muscle biopsy or genetic testing is required for confirmative diagnosis.[6,12,17]

MANAGEMENT

Only after a thorough history and examination that rules out potential causes of toe walking can ITW be diagnosed. Williams and colleagues[36] developed an online Toe Walking Tool that was designed to help primary care providers assess pediatric toe walkers and determine if a diagnosis of ITW (**Table 1**). The Toe Walking Tool is a systematic method of assessment and questions to determine if the child in question is healthy or if further evaluation or referral is warranted.

For children younger than 2 years who present for initial evaluation with chief complaint of toe walking without an Achilles contracture, it is recommended that no formal intervention be performed and that observation is the best management. Often, children will begin improvement in their gait after 2 to 3 years of age.

If a child does have a contracture of the Achilles or is older than 2 years, treatment can be recommended. Stretching of the plantar flexors and strengthening of the dorsiflexors with physical therapy and with a home exercise program is often the first line of treatment. Night splinting is also often recommended. Occupational therapy referral may be beneficial if the provider feels that there is a sensory component to the patient's toe walking.

If children do not respond to initial conservative management, serial casting to stretch the Achilles can be initiated with or without the concurrent utilization of botulinum type A (Botox) injections.[37] Trained physical therapists, physical medicine and rehabilitation physicians, or orthopedic surgeons that specialize in pediatrics can complete serial casting. There are mixed results regarding improved outcomes with using Botox injections in conjunction with serial casting, with the greatest improvements often being seen CP patients that toe walk.[37–39] Serial casting is often the most beneficial of nonsurgical treatment options to increase range of motion in toe

Table 1
Toe Walking Tool questions and order of progression

Question	Theme	Response that May Indicate a Medical Cause
Name	Demographics	N/A
Date of birth	Demographics	N/A
Gender	Demographics	N/A
Does the child toe walk	Demographics	N/A
Does the child have a condition that you have sought medical assistance for and/or been diagnosed with a condition causing the toe walking?	Demographics	N/A
Does the child have a diagnosis of autism spectrum disorder?	Neurogenic	Yes
Does the child have a diagnosis of cerebral palsy?	Neuromuscular	Yes
Does the child have a diagnosis of muscular dystrophy?	Neuromuscular	Yes
Does the child's family have a history of muscular dystrophy?	Neuromuscular	Yes
Does the child have a diagnosis of global developmental delay?	Neurogenic	Yes
When the child was born, was their birth weight over 2500 g?	Neuromuscular	No
When the child was born were they over 37 wk gestation?	Neuromuscular	No
Was the child admitted to special needs nursery/neonatal intensive care after birth?	Neuromuscular	Yes
Did the child independently walk prior to 20 mo of age?	Neuromuscular/neurogenic	No
Does the child have a family member that toe walks with no other medical condition?	Demographic	N/A
Does the child toe walk on one foot only?	Traumatic	Yes
Is the child toe walking in response to pain?	Traumatic	Yes
Did the child previously walk flat footed and only recently start to toe walk?	Traumatic/neuromuscular	Yes
When you ask the child to walk on their heels are they able to?	Traumatic/neuromuscular	No
On testing the ankle or hamstring range of motion is there a clonus and/or catch?	Neuromuscular	No
When asking the child to get up from the floor is there a positive Gower's sign?	Neuromuscular	Yes

(continued on next page)

Table 1
(continued)

Question	Theme	Response that May Indicate a Medical Cause
Is there a normal knee jerk reflex?	Neuromuscular	No
Is there a normal Babinski reflex?	Neuromuscular	No
Are the hip flexors tight for the child's age (Thomas test)? Are the hamstrings tight for the child's age (popliteal angle)? Is the gastrocnemius and soleus tight for the child's age (lunge test)?	Neuromuscular	Answer of Yes for 2 of the questions
Does the child have more than 2 significant delayed developmental milestones?	Neurogenic	Yes
Does the child have limited eye contact, have strict rituals or ritual-related behaviors, such as lining up toys, rocking, or spinning?	Neurogenic	Yes

From Williams CM, Tinley P, Curtin M. The Toe Walking Tool: a novel method for assessing idiopathic toe walking children. Gait & Posture 2010;32:509; with permission.

walkers with decreased ankle range of motion, and therefore, is strongly recommended before surgical intervention.[12,13,40] Botox injections have also been used in combination with an exercise program, with demonstrated improvement in gait but limited cessation of toe walking.[41] After serial casting is completed, the child should be fitted for an orthosis to maintain any gains made from the casting. Although custom ankle-foot orthoses are most often prescribed, as they control the ankle and limit the ability for toe walking, less restrictive foot orthoses may be more accepted by children and their families, therefore, potentially increasing compliance, and can be trialed initially.[42] Compliance with home exercise stretching programs and use of splints are necessary to maintain correction.

Specialist Referrals

Children with a diagnosis of idiopathic toe walking can often be treated appropriately by a primary care provider with observation or referrals to physical or occupational therapy, especially those who are younger than 3 years, are without decreased range of ankle motion, and those for whom there is no concern for an underlying cause of the toe walking. Referrals to specialists should be made when there is muscular atrophy, an abnormal neurologic examination, unilateral toe walking without a known neurologic diagnosis, or development of new-onset toe walking after a previously established gait. Referrals to specialists should be considered for patients with persistent toe walking and for patients with decreased range of motion of the ankle.

Referring a toe walker to a pediatric orthopedic surgeon is recommended when there is persistent toe walking past the age of 3 and decreased range of motion of the ankle. If conservative treatments were attempted but failed, or children have a fixed equinus contracture, surgical intervention is often warranted and has been shown to have beneficial results.[4,6,27,43] Children with diagnosed CP may also benefit from referral to a pediatric orthopedic surgeon for gait evaluation and possible surgical management for contractures. Surgical options may include tendo-Achilles lengthening, gastrocnemius recession, and a possible tibialis anterior or posterior transfer if the patient has concomitant hindfoot varus.

Patients presenting with acute or progressive toe walking, those with clonus or abnormal neurologic examinations, or those with concerns for weakness should have further testing, most often an MRI of the brain or spine, and be referred to a pediatric neurologist or neurosurgeon. Potentially, lesions of the spine or brain may also be malignant, and referral to oncology may also be warranted.

For any child with persistent ITW, screening for autism should be completed, and further evaluation should be made by a developmental pediatrician, as ITW has been found to be a marker for developmental delays and autism.[7,21]

DISCUSSION

There is debate regarding the most appropriate management of children with ITW because of limited long-term studies on the natural history of toe walkers.[44] Although some studies find that many patients will grow out of ITW or have improved gait, other studies find that patients may instead compensate for their plantar flexor contractures with out-toeing and may subsequently have decreased ankle range of motion, fixed contractures of their Achilles, or deformities of their lower extremities such as external tibial torsion or forefoot splay.[1,3,5,25,27,32,43] Eiff and colleagues[45] published in 2006 that evidence-based research recommends against serial casting and surgery in the management of children with ITW, as observation alone can result in similar levels of decreased frequency of toe walking at follow-up. Bullying and other neuropsychiatric manifestations should also be a consideration with older children and teenagers that are toe walkers.[46]

Most important for the medical provider evaluating the toe-walking child is to determine if there is an underlying cause for the toe walking, which should be treated or referred for appropriate management. For those children with true ITW after other diagnoses have been ruled out, it may be most appropriate to have a discussion with the family regarding treatment options and potential outcomes. Dietz and Khunsree[47] recommend considering ITW as a cosmetic deformity that only requires treatment if it bothers the child or the family.[47] The family and the provider should together create appropriate realistic goals and then determine the best plan for the child.

REFERENCES

1. Sala DA, Shulman LH, Kennedy RF, et al. Idiopathic toe-walking: a review. Dev Med Child Neurol 1999;41(12):846–8.
2. Williams CM, Michalitsis J, Murphy A, et al. Do external stimuli impact the gait of children with idiopathic toe walking? A study protocol for a within-subject randomised control trial. BMJ Open 2013;3:e0002389.
3. Schoenecker PL, Rich MM. The lower extremity. In: Morrisy RT, Weinstein SL, editors. Lovell and winter's pediatric orthopaedics. 6th edition. Philadelphia: Lippincott Williams & Wilkins; 2006. p. 1204–6. Chapter 28.
4. Hall JE, Salter RB, Bhalla SK. Congenital short tendo calcaneus. J Bone Joint Surg Br 1967;49:695–7.
5. Hirsch G, Wagner B. The natural history of idiopathic toe walking: a long-term follow up of fourteen conservatively treated children. Acta Paediatr 2004;93: 196–9.

6. Oetgen ME, Peden S. Idiopathic toe walking. J Am Acad Orthop Surg 2012;20: 292–300.

7. Shulman LH, Sala DA, Chu MY, et al. Developmental implications of idiopathic toe walking. J Pediatr 1997;130(4):541–6.

8. Montgomery P, Gauger J. Sensory dysfunction in children who toe walk. Phys Ther 1978;58(10):1195–204.

9. Williams CM, Tinley P, Cutin M, et al. Is idiopathic toe walking really idiopathic? The motor skills and sensory processing abilities associated with idiopathic toe walking gait. J Child Neurol 2014;29(1):71–8.

10. Eastwood DM, Dennett X, Shield LK, et al. Muscle abnormalities in idiopathic toe walkers. J Pediatr Orthop B 1997;6(3):215–8.

11. Engelbert R, Gorter JW, Uiterwaal C, et al. Idiopathic toe-walking in children, adolescents and young adults: a matter of local or generalised stiffness? BMC Musculoskelet Disord 2011;12:61.

12. Fox A, Deakin S, Pettigrew G, et al. Serial casting in the treatment of idiopathic toe-walkers and a review of the literature. Acta Orthop Belg 2006;72(6):722–30.

13. Engstrom P, Tedroff K. The prevalence and course of idiopathic toe-walking in 5-year-old children. Pediatrics 2012;130(2):279–84.

14. Karol LA. Disorders of the brain. In: Herring JA, editor. Tachdjian's pediatric orthopaedics. 4th edition. Philadelphia: Saunders/Elsevier; 2008. p. 1277–396. Chapter 25.

15. Pernet J, Billiaux A, Auvin S, et al. Early onset toe-walking in toddlers: a cause for concern? J Pediatr 2010;157(3):496–8.

16. McDonald CM. Clinical approach to the diagnostic evaluation of hereditary and acquired neuromuscular diseases. Phys Med Rehabil Clin N Am 2012;23(3): 495–563.

17. Hosalkar HS, Moroz LA, Drummond DS, et al. Neuromuscular disorders of infancy and childhood arthrogryposis. In: Dorman JP, editor. Pediatric orthopedics: core knowledge in orthopedics. 1st edition. Philadelphia: Elsevier Mosby; 2005. p. 454–82. Chapter 18.

18. Frick SL. Normal growth and development in pediatric orthopedics. In: Dorman JP, editor. Pediatric orthopedics: core knowledge in orthopedics. 1st edition. Philadelphia: Elsevier Mosby; 2005. p. 1–14. Chapter 1.

19. Accardo PJ, Morrow J, Heaney MS, et al. Toe walking and language development. Clin Pediatr 1992;31:158–60.

20. Accardo PJ, Whitman BY. Toe walking: a marker for language disorders in the developmentally disabled. Clin Pediatr 1989;28:347–50.

21. Barrow WJ, Jaworski M, Accardo PJ. Persistent toe walking in autism. J Child Neurol 2011;26(5):619–21.

22. Stone WL, Lee EB, Ashford L, et al. Can autism be diagnosed accurately in children under 3 years? J Child Psychol Psychiatry 1999;40:219–26.

23. Baber S, Michalitsis J, Fahey M, et al. A comparison of the birth characteristics of idiopathic toe walking and toe walking gait due to medical reasons. J Pediatr 2016;171:290–3.

24. Gerber RJ, Wilks T, Erdie-Lalena C. Developmental milestones: motor development. 2015. Available at: http://pedsinreview.aappublications.org/content/31/7/267. Accessed December 28, 2015.

25. Sobel E, Caselli MA, Velez Z. Effect of persistent toe walking on ankle equinus. Analysis of 60 idiopathic toe walkers. J Am Podiatr Med Assoc 1997;87(1):17–22.

26. Clark E, Sweeney JK, Yocum A, et al. Effects of motor control intervention for children with idiopathic toe walking: a 5-case series. Pediatr Phys Thor 2010;22(4): 417–26.

27. Stricker SJ, Angulo JC. Idiopathic toe walking: a comparison of treatment methods. J Pediatr Orthop 1998;18(3):289–93.

28. Sabharwal S, Kumar A. Methods for assessing leg length discrepancy. Clin Orthop Relat Res 2008;466(12):2910–22.

29. Beebe AC, Kerpsack JM. Pediatric musculoskeletal examination. In: Dorman JP, editor. Pediatric orthopedics: core knowledge in orthopedics. 1st edition. Philadelphia: Elsevier Mosby; 2005. p. 14–35. Chapter 2.

30. Katz K, Rosenthal A, Yosipovitch Z. Normal ranges of popliteal angle in children. J Pediatr Orthop 1992;12(2):229–31.

31. Caselli MA. Habitual toe walking. Podiatry Management 2002;163–78.

32. Hicks R, Durinick N, Gage JR. Differentiation of idiopathic toe-walking and cerebral palsy. J Pediatr Orthop 1988;8:160–3.

33. Westberry DE, Davids JR, Davis RB, et al. Idiopathic toe walking: a kinematic and kinetic profile. J Pediatr Orthop 2008;28(3):352–8.

34. Kalen V, Adler N, Bleck EE. Electromyography of idiopathic toe walking. J Pediatr Orthop 1986;6(3):31–3.

35. Griffen PP, Wheelhouse WW, Shiavi R, et al. Habitual toe-walkers: a clinical and electromyographic gait analysis. J Bone Joint Surg Am 1977;59:97–101.

36. Williams CM, Tinley P, Curtin M. The toe walking tool: a novel method for assessing idiopathic toe walking children. Gait Posture 2010;32:508–11.

37. Brunt D, Woo R, Kim HD, et al. Effect of botulinum toxin type A on gait of children who are idiopathic toe walkers. J Surg Orthop Adv 2004;13:149–55.

38. Jacks LK, Michels DM, Smith BP, et al. Clinical usefulness of botulinum toxin in the lower extremity. Foot Ankle Clin 2004;9:339–48.

39. Kay RM, Rethlefsen SA, Fern-Buneo A, et al. Botulinum toxin as an adjunct to serial casting treatment in children with cerebral palsy. J Bone Joint Surg Am 2004; 86-A(11):2377–84.

40. Katz MM, Mubarak SJ. Hereditary tendo achilles contractures. J Pediatr Orthop 1984;4(6):711–4.

41. Engstrom P, Gutierrez-Farewik EM, Bartonek A, et al. Does botulinum toxin A improve the walking pattern in children with idiopathic toe walking? J Child Orthop 2010;4(4):301–8.

42. Herrin K, Geil M. A comparison of orthoses in the treatment of idiopathic toe walking: a randomized control trial. Prosthet Orthot Int 2016;40(2):262–9.

43. Eastwood DM, Menelaus MB, Dickens DRV, et al. Idiopathic toe-walking: does treatment alter the natural history? J Pediatr Orthop B 2000;9:47–9.

44. van Kuijk AAA, Kosters R, Vugts M, et al. Treatment for idiopathic toe walking: a systematic review of the literature. J Rehabil Med 2014;46:945–57.

45. Eiff PM, Steiner E, Judkins DZ. What is the appropriate evaluation and treatment of children who are "toe walkers"? J Fam Pract 2006;55(5):447–50.

46. Engstrom P, Van't Hooft I, Tedroff K. Neuropsychiatric symptoms and problems among children with idiopathic toe walking. J Pediatr Orthop 2012;32:848–52.

47. Dietz F, Khunsree S. Idiopathic toe walking: to treat or not to treat, that is the question. Iowa Orthop J 2012;32:184–8.

Immunization Update

Chris Barry, PA-C, MMSc

KEYWORDS

- Vaccines • Immunizations • Pediatrics • Vaccine schedule • Infant vaccines
- Vaccine hesitancy

KEY POINTS

- Vaccines are essential tools in disease prevention. Vaccines have saved countless lives, and they should continue to be used to the greatest extent possible.
- Physician assistants (PAs) must be familiar with vaccine myths and the truth behind each myth.
- The current immunization schedule and catch-up schedule as well as a list of reputable sources of vaccine information must be readily available as patient handouts.
- PAs must make strong, same-day recommendations for vaccines.

INTRODUCTION

Since their introduction, vaccines have arguably been the most successful and important methods to prevent disease in the history of modern medicine.[1,2] Because PAs are trained on the importance of preventive health care, vaccines are the ultimate tools in their arsenal. This article reviews how vaccines have benefitted (and continue to benefit) children, including information on each vaccine currently recommended for children and the diseases they prevent. Common myths about vaccines also are discussed, along with refutations to each myth. Finally, strategies for establishing and maintaining a successful vaccination program are discussed.

Vaccines have been responsible for reducing and eliminating several deadly and debilitating diseases that were once commonplace. **Table 1** shows the impressive decreases in various diseases since introduction of vaccines. Yet despite the reductions in morbidity and mortality, not enough children are immunized. The most recent National Immunization Survey (NIS) shows that a high percentage of kindergarten students are up to date on their immunizations but the NIS-Teen survey shows there is significant room for improvement in immunization rates among teens and preteens.[3,4]

Disclosures: Advisory Board, Merck Vaccines, US HPV Advisory Board; Speaker's Bureau, Merck Vaccines, HPV Vaccine.
Jeffers, Mann, & Artman Pediatrics, 2406 Blue Ridge Rd., Suite 100, Raleigh, NC 27607, USA
E-mail address: cmbarry@gmail.com

Physician Assist Clin 1 (2016) 615–625
http://dx.doi.org/10.1016/j.cpha.2016.05.007
2405-7991/16/© 2016 Elsevier Inc. All rights reserved.

Table 1
Comparison of prevaccine and current reported morbidity of vaccine-preventable diseases and vaccine adverse events, United States

Disease	Prevaccine Era[a]	2015	Decrease (%)
Diphtheria	175,885	0	100
Measles	503,282	188	>99
Mumps	152,209	29	>99
Pertussis	147,271	992	>99
Polio (paralytic)	16,316	0	100
Rubella	47,745	2	>99
Tetanus	1314	1	>99
Hib and unknown (<5 y)	20,000[b]	148	>99

[a] Baseline twentieth-century annual morbidity.
[b] Estimated because no national reporting existed in the prevaccine era.
From Roush, SW, Murphy, TV. Historical comparisons of morbidity and mortality for vaccine-preventable diseases in the United States. JAMA 2007;298(18):2155–2163.

CHILDHOOD IMMUNIZATIONS AND THE DISEASES THEY PREVENT
Hepatitis B

According to the Centers for Disease Control and Prevention (CDC), 2000 to 4000 people die in the United States from cirrhosis or liver cancer caused by hepatitis B. Hepatitis B can be spread by vertical transmission from mother to baby. Hepatitis B can also be spread from direct contact with blood or bodily fluids and can survive for over a week outside the body. The hepatitis B vaccine is recommended for all children to be completed in the first year of life.

Diphtheria, Tetanus, and Pertussis

The diphtheria and tetanus toxoids and acellular pertussis vaccine (DTaP) and tetanus toxoid, reduced diphtheria toxoid, and acellular pertussis (Tdap) vaccines protect infants, children, and young adults against diphtheria, tetanus, and pertussis. Diphtheria is an acute communicable respiratory illness caused by Corynebacterium diphtheriae, which causes disease by releasing toxins and has a mortality rate of 5% to 10% in older children and adults and up to 20% in children under age 5.[5] Symptoms of diphtheria are often similar to those of an upper respiratory infection, but there is frequently a thick membranous coating on the posterior pharynx, which can cause dyspnea and dysphagia.

Tetanus is a central nervous system disorder caused by toxins produced by the anaerobic bacteria Clostridium tetani. These bacteria are commonly found in soil as well as feces from animals and humans. They enter the human body through a puncture wound or other traumatic injury. Symptoms of tetanus include trismus—muscle spasms usually beginning in the jaw muscles (hence the nickname, lockjaw), followed by neck stiffness, dysphagia, and rigidity of the abdominal muscles. Fever, tachycardia, diaphoresis, and hypertension may follow. Muscle spasms may last for several minutes and may continue for weeks to months.

Pertussis, also known as whooping cough, is an acute respiratory illness caused by the bacteria Bordetella pertussis. Pertussis presents differently in infants and adolescents. The classic presentation, most commonly seen in infants and young children, includes paroxysms of cough, followed by an inspiratory whoop and often post-tussive vomiting.[6] The inspiratory whoop and post-tussive vomiting are seen most commonly in infants less than 1 year old.[7] In older children and adolescents, pertussis can be difficult to detect. These children may be asymptomatic or have only a mild illness without classic pertussis symptoms.[8] Overall mortality from pertussis is low but is highest among infants under 2 months of age, especially those infants born prematurely.[9]

Due to waning immunity and suboptimal vaccination rates, there have been several recent outbreaks in the United States. The Tdap vaccine is recommended for all 11 to 12 year olds for prevention of pertussis. Currently, there is no recommendation for a pertussis booster, despite some evidence suggesting waning immunity against pertussis.[10] The only exception is that Tdap is recommended to be given to pregnant women with each pregnancy.[11]

Haemophilus Influenzae Type B

Prior to widespread immunization, *Haemophilus influenzae* type B (Hib) infection was a common cause of invasive bacterial infections, including meningitis, epiglottitis, pneumonia, and bacteremia. After introduction of the Hib conjugate vaccine in the 1990s, Hib disease was virtually eliminated in the United States.[12] Hib vaccine is seeing widespread use in Asia and Eastern Europe, with a dramatic impact on disease incidence and effective prevention of pneumonia and bacterial meningitis.[13]

Polio

Infection with poliovirus was widespread and devastating at one time. Polio has been eliminated, however, from the United States and most parts of the world due to the success of the polio vaccine. The last case of wild-type polio in the United States was prior to 1980, but because there are still small pockets of polio scattered throughout the world, polio vaccination continues to be recommended in the United States.[14]

Rotavirus

Prior to the introduction of rotavirus vaccines, rotavirus was a leading cause of severe gastroenteritis in infants and children.[15] Initial rotavirus vaccines were recalled due to a slightly increased rate of intussusception. The current rotavirus vaccines on the market did not show an increase in intussusception and have been highly effective in reducing rotavirus disease. These vaccines have reduced rotavirus-related emergency department visits and hospitalizations by more than 95%.[16]

Pneumococcal Vaccine

Streptococcus pneumoniae (pneumococcus) is a major cause of bacterial pneumonia, sepsis, and meningitis, mainly in children less than 2 years of age. The pneumococcal conjugate vaccine used in the United States is responsible for a significant decrease in invasive pneumococcal disease, due to both direct protection and herd immunity.[17] The 7-valent pneumococcal conjugate vaccine was replaced by a 13-valent version in 2010, providing even broader protection against invasive pneumococcal disease.[18]

Measles, Mumps, and Rubella

Measles is a highly contagious virus, spread by respiratory droplets, and characterized by a fever, malaise, cough, conjunctivitis, and a distinct rash that starts around the hairline, moves to the face and neck, and proceeds down the body. Since the widespread use of measles vaccination, global measles deaths have decreased by 96% from the prevaccine era.[19] Sporadic outbreaks of measles in the United States have occurred in recent years, underscoring the importance of continued immunization.

Mumps, another viral illness, is less contagious than measles, and is generally a mild disease in children, although it can be more serious in adults. Mumps is often responsible for cases of parotitis and orchitis. Prior to routine vaccination, however, mumps was a leading cause of viral meningitis and a common cause of hearing loss in children.[20] With routine vaccination against mumps, the number of cases of mumps decreased by 99%.[21]

Rubella, or German measles, is a virus spread through respiratory droplets. Clinical manifestations are generally mild and include a rash; however, up to half of people infected with rubella virus are asymptomatic. The most serious complications of rubella involve damage to the fetus, causing miscarriage and birth defects, including congenital rubella syndrome (hearing impairment, congenital heart defects, cataracts, and glaucoma).[22]

Varicella

Varicella-zoster virus (VZV) is a highly contagious virus that causes chickenpox and shingles (herpes zoster). VZV is causes a vesicular rash, along with fever, malaise, and loss of appetite. The virus can also cause central nervous system complications, including encephalitis and Reye syndrome.[23] Since the identification of aspirin as a major cause of Reye syndrome in varicella patients, however, most patients are instructed to avoid aspirin when febrile; as a result, Reye syndrome is extremely rare.[24] VZV is typically more severe in adults.

Hepatitis A

Hepatitis A is a viral illness that is spread most commonly through fecal-oral transmission. Most cases of hepatitis A are self-limited, but hepatitis A occasionally causes acute liver failure (<1% of cases).[25] Although hepatitis A is more prevalent in South America, Africa, and Asia, it is still a common disease in the United States. Cases of hepatitis A have decreased approximately 30-fold in the United States since children were routinely vaccinated against hepatitis A beginning in 1999.[26]

Meningococcal Vaccines

Meningitis caused by *Neisseria meningitidis* can be rapidly fatal, causing death in the matter of hours if not treated properly. Vaccines to prevent meningitis caused by this bacteria have been successful at preventing morbidity and mortality in children and young adults. Meningitis outbreaks often afflict college freshman living in dormitories.[27] Vaccines that prevent meningococcal serogroups A, C, Y, and W135 are recommended for all 11-year-old to 12 year-old children, with additional recommendations for younger children who are at greater risk for meningitis. A booster dose at age 16 is also recommended.[28]

Vaccines to prevent serogroup B, which is responsible for approximately 32% of bacterial meningitis cases, were introduced into the United States in 2015.[29]

According to the Advisory Committee on Immunization Practices (ACIP), meningococcal B vaccines should be given to those with complement deficiency or asplenia, travelers to countries where meningitis B is endemic, and those living in areas with a meningitis disease outbreak caused by another serogroup of meningitis. The meningococcal B vaccine may also be given to 16 to 23 year olds for short-term protection against serogroup B meningitis (permissive recommendation), but the ACIP stopped short of routinely recommneding the meningococcal B vaccine.[30]

Human Papillomavirus

Human papillomavirus (HPV) is a virus that is spread through intimate contact. Intercourse is not necessary, but it is the most common form of transmission of HPV.[31] HPV is extremely prevalent among sexually active people. It is estimated that 80% of sexually active women are been infected with HPV by age 50. More than 120 HPV types have been identified. Many are low risk, but the high-risk types have been detected in 99% of cervical cancers.[31] Most HPV infections are asymptomatic and result in no clinical symptoms or disease. Most HPV infections resolve spontaneously, but a small percentage of infected people develops persistent infection.[32] For HPV-related cervical disease, it is difficult to predict which patients with infection or abnormal cytology will progress to clinically significant disease versus spontaneously regress.[33]

A new study showed that the HPV vaccine is already positively affecting HPV infection rates. Among girls ages 14 to 19, rates of infection with the 4 HPV types included in the quadrivalent HPV vaccine decreased from 11.5% to 4.3%. The same study also showed that among 14-year-old to 24 year-old adolescents and women who were sexually active, rates of HPV infection with the HPV types contained in the quadrivalent HPV vaccine was 2.1% among those who were vaccinated versus 16.9% among those who were not vaccinated.[34]

HPV vaccines are highly effective in preventing the HPV types contained in the vaccines. The vaccines prevent cancers and precancers in both males and females. Clinical trials showed higher antibody titers amount younger participants (ages 9–15) than in older participants (16 and older). For these reasons, and because of the importance of vaccinating before potential exposure to HPV, the HPV vaccine is routinely recommended for both genders at age 11 to 12, with catch-up dosing for older children.

Influenza

Every year, influenza (flu), a seasonal respiratory virus, occurs in outbreaks, typically during the winter. Generally, influenza is a self-limited disease, but in children with weakened immune systems and certain respiratory conditions, flu can have significant morbidity and mortality. Even in otherwise healthy children, there is a risk of hospitalization and even death from influenza. Between 2004 and 2012, 830 flu-related pediatric deaths were reported, and of those whose medical history was known, 43% did not have a high-risk medical condition.[35]

Flu vaccine is recommended for all children aged 6 months and older. For children over 2, the injectable or intranasal flu vaccine may be given; for children less than 2, only the injectable flu vaccine may be given. In all cases, flu vaccine must be given annually to afford the best protection. There are still many myths surrounding the flu vaccine that are discussed later (**Box 1**).

Box 1
Common vaccine myths

- Vaccines overwhelm the immune system
- MMR vaccine causes autism
- Thimerosal causes autism
- Flu vaccine causes flu
- HPV vaccine leads to earlier sexual debut or risky sexual behavior

---

VACCINE MYTHS AND TRUTHS
The Antivaccine Movement

There is certainly an abundance of useful, factual vaccine information on the Internet (**Box 2**). There is also a lot of misinformation, however, on the Internet that can look factual. For example, the Web site entitled, "National Vaccine Information Center" (www.nvic.org), is actually a cover for an antivaccine Web site, run largely by people who are not in the medical field.[36]

Vaccines have become victims of their own success, because many parents have never seen many of the illnesses that are vaccinated against. As health care providers, PAs know how critically important vaccines are for the health of our patients. Many parents make their vaccine decisions, however, based on conjecture, social media postings, and misinformation. To improve immunization rates, PAs need to understand some of the common misconceptions parents have about vaccines and must be ready to counter misinformation with truths.

MYTH: VACCINES OVERWHELM THE IMMUNE SYSTEM
Truth

When infants are given the recommended series of vaccines at their well-child visits, a common parental concern is that too many vaccines are given at one time and will overwhelm the immune system. Although infants do receive more vaccines than in years past, this serves to protect children against many more diseases than in the past.

Box 2
Immunization resources

For Parents and Clinicians

http://www.immunize.org

Vaccine information for patients and professionals, lots of easy to find information on vaccines and vaccine-preventable diseases, current vaccine information statements (VIS) in a variety of languages, and articles for parents and clinicians

http://www.chop.edu/vec

Children's Hospital of Philadelphia Vaccine Information Center

http://www.cdc.gov/vaccines/

Excellent vaccine information and disease epidemiology

https://www.healthychildren.org/English/safety-prevention/immunizations/Pages/default.aspx

Health Children Immunization information

For Clinicians

http://www.cdc.gov/vaccines/hcp/conversations/index.html

Resources for addressing vaccine-hesitant parents and patients

http://www2.aap.org/immunization/pediatricians/communicating.html AAP Immunization: Resources for Clinicians for Vaccine Conversations

It is estimated that an infant's immune system is capable of handling approximately 10,000 antigens at once.[37]

Therefore, the immunizations that are routinely given only use 0.1% of the capacity of the immune system. Young infants have an enormous capacity to handle multiple vaccines at once as well as other environmental challenges. Compared with the challenges the immune system is exposed to on a daily basis, the challenge from the components in vaccines is miniscule. The number of antigens infants are exposed to today is far fewer than in the 1960s and 1980s, primarily due to the switch from whole-cell pertussis (which contained approximately 3000 antigens) to acellular pertussis vaccine (which contains 2–5 antigens).[37]

MYTH: MEASLES, MUMPS, AND RUBELLA VACCINE CAUSES AUTISM
Truth

The measles, mumps, and rubella (MMR) vaccine does not cause autism. A causal association between the MMR vaccine and autism has never been shown in scientific literature. Furthermore, there are no plausible biological mechanisms by which this vaccine could cause autism or any other developmental delays.

Dr Andrew Wakefield, a British physician who published an article in *The Lancet* in 1998, purported a link between the MMR vaccine and autism.[38] The article was retracted in 2010, amid cries of poor science. In 2011, the study was exposed as fraudulent and shown to demonstrate a conflict of interest, because Wakefield stood to gain financially from a lawsuit against a vaccine manufacturer.[39]

MYTH: THIMEROSAL CAUSES AUTISM

The preservative thimerosal contains approximately 49% ethyl mercury. Ethyl mercury is chemically very different from methyl mercury, which is a product of industrial processes. The ethyl mercury found in thimerosal is removed from the bloodstream much faster than methyl mercury, and ethyl mercury does not cross the blood-brain barrier due to its molecular size. Because of the short half-life of ethyl mercury, it does not accumulate in the body or cause autism.[40] In addition, clinical features of mercury poisoning are significantly different from autism. In 1999, largely in response to parental concerns that thimerosal in vaccines could potentially be responsible for autism, thimerosal was removed from most vaccines. In 2001, all vaccines contained either no thimerosal or trace amounts of thimerosal with the exception of some multidose flu vials. Several studies have been performed, all of which have shown no causal link between thimerosal and autism. Autism rates have risen despite the removal of thimerosal.[41–44]

MYTH: THE FLU VACCINE CAUSES THE FLU, OR "I DO NOT NEED THE FLU VACCINE"

Despite scientific evidence to the contrary, 43% of Americans believe the flu vaccine can cause the flu.[45] The flu shot is composed of inactivated or recombinant flu virus, so it is impossible that the vaccine can give patients the flu. The nasal spray flu vaccine cannot give anyone the flu either. The nasal flu vaccine is a live attenuated vaccine that is cold adapted, so it can survive in the nose but cannot cause infection in warmer parts of the body, such as the lungs.

MYTH: HUMAN PAPILLOMAVIRUS (HPV) VACCINE CAUSES CHILDREN TO BE SEXUALLY ACTIVE AT AN EARLIER AGE AND/OR PROMOTES RISKIER SEXUAL BEHAVIOR AMONG TEENAGERS, AND/OR "MY CHILD DOES NOT NEED THAT VACCINE BECAUSE SHE/HE WILL NOT EVER BE EXPOSED TO HPV VACCINE"

As with all vaccines, the HPV vaccine must be given prior to any exposure to HPV to be most effective. HPV can be passed even when the infected person has no symptoms, making it that much harder to control. By immunizing children against HPV routinely at age 11 to 12 years, an HPV-naïve patient population is ensured. To address parental fears that the HPV vaccine leads to promiscuity or risky sexual behavior among teens, Liddon and colleagues[46] showed that administering the HPV vaccine does NOT encourage sexual promiscuity. This study showed that, among 15 year-old to 24-year-old female patients, HPV vaccination was not associated with being sexually active or with the total number of lifetime sex partners.[46]

STRATEGIES FOR SUCCESSFUL VACCINATION

With the increasing amount of antivaccine sentiment, despite valid scientific evidence proving the success of vaccines, it is important for PAs and other pediatric health care providers to take a stand for what is best for children. A successful immunization program must be a team effort, from the people who schedule appointments, to the check-in receptionist, to the nurse/medical assistant, to the provider. Immunizations are most commonly given at well-child visits but can also be given at non–well-child visits to further increase the number of vaccinees.

Providers should also be able to provide a list of resources on various vaccines to their patients. A list of some helpful Web sites is in **Box 2**. One of the biggest predictors of whether a child will receive a vaccine at the visit is a strong, same-day recommendation by the clinician.[47] Research has confirmed that this presumptive approach has resulted in a higher rate of immunization versus the participatory approach, where there is more parental decision-making latitude.[48] Health care providers must take the time to educate patients and their families about vaccines. The following are recommendations to increase the chances patients will receive their immunizations on time:

Know which vaccines are recommended for each age group and why (See CDC-recommended immunization schedule for persons 0 through 18 years old, united states, 2016. Available at: http://www.cdc.gov/vaccines/schedules/hcp/imz/child-adolescent.html.)

- Learn the arguments that antivaccine alarmists are using, and use the scientific truth to educate parents.
- Take time to dispel vaccine myths.
- Direct parents to Web sites of reputable sources of information.
- Look for ways to increase vaccine opportunities, including giving vaccines at non–well-check visits.
- Provide a strong, simple, same-day recommendation for vaccination.

REFERENCES

1. Centers for Disease Control and Prevention (CDC). Ten great public health achievements – United States, 1900-1999. MMWR Morb Mortal Wkly Rep 1999; 48(12):241–3.

2. Jagessar N, Lazarus JV, Laurent E, et al. Immunization: mind the gap. Vaccine 2008;26(52):6736–7.

3. Seither R, Calhoun K, Knighton CL, et al. Vaccination coverage among children in kindergarten-United States, 2014-15 school year. MMWR Morb Mortal Wkly Rep 2015;64(33):897–904.

4. Reagan-Steiner S, Yankey D, Jeyarajah J, et al. National, regional, state, and selected local area vaccination coverage among adolescents aged 13-17 years–United States, 2014. MMWR Morb Mortal Wkly Rep 2015;64(29): 784–92.

5. Centers for Disease Control and Prevention. Diphtheria. In: Hamborsky J, Kroger A, Wolfe S, editors. Epidemiology and prevention of vaccine-preventable diseases. The pink book: course textbook. 13th edition. Washington, DC: Public Health Foundation; 2015. p. 107–18.

6. Mattoo S, Cherry JD. Molecular pathogenesis, epidemiology, and clinical manifestations of respiratory infections due to Bordetella pertussis and other Bordetella subspecies. Clin Microbiol Rev 2005;18(2):326.

7. Chan MH, Ma L, Sidelinger D, et al. The California pertussis epidemic 2010: a review of 986 pediatric case reports from San Diego county. J Pediatric Infect Dis Soc 2012;1:47.

8. Ward JI, Cherry JD, Chang SJ, et al. Bordetella Pertussis infections in vaccinated and unvaccinated adolescents and adults, as assessed in a national prospective randomized Acellular Pertussis Vaccine Trial (APERT). Clin Infect Dis 2006;43(2): 151–7.

9. Mikelova LK, Halperin SA, Scheifele D, et al. Predictors of death in infants hospitalized with pertussis: a case-control study of 16 pertussis deaths in Canada. J Pediatr 2003;143(5):576.

10. Broder KR, Cortese MM, Iskander JK, et al. Preventing tetanus, diphtheria, and pertussis among adolescents: use of tetanus toxoid, reduced diphtheria toxoid and acellular pertussis vaccines. MMWR Recomm Rep 2006; 55(RR03):1–34.

11. American College of Obstetricians and Gynecologists Committee Opinion No. 566: update on immunization and pregnancy: tetanus, diphtheria, and pertussis vaccination. Obstet Gynecol 2013;121:1411–4.

12. Wenger JD. Epidemiology of Haemophilus influenzae type b disease and impact of Haemophilus influenzae type b conjugate vaccines in the United States and Canada. Pediatr Infect Dis J 1998;17:S132–6.

13. Hajjeh R, Mulholland K, Schuchat A, et al. Progress towards demonstrating the impact of Haemophilus influenzae type b conjugate vaccines globally. J Pediatr 2013;163(1):S1–3.

14. Kim-Farley RJ, Bart KJ, Schonberger LB, et al. Poliomyelitis in the USA: virtual elimination of disease caused by wild virus. Lancet 1984;2(8415): 1315.

15. Cortese MM, Parashar UD. Prevention of rotavirus gastroenteritis among infants and children: recommendations of the Advisory Committee on Immunization Practices (ACIP). MMWR Recomm Rep 2009;58(RR-2):1.

16. Vesikari T, Matson DO, Dennehy P, et al. Safety and efficacy of a pentavalent human–bovine (WC3) reassortant rotavirus vaccine. N Engl J Med 2006;354(1): 23–33.

17. Talbot TR, Poehling KA, Hartert TV, et al. Reduction in high rates of antibiotic-nonsusceptible invasive pneumococcal disease in tennessee after

introduction of the pneumococcal conjugate vaccine. Clin Infect Dis 2004; 39(5):641.

18. Moore MR, Link-Gelles R, Schaffner W, et al. Effect of use of 13-valent pneumococcal conjugate vaccine in children on invasive pneumococcal disease in children and adults in the USA: analysis of multisite, population-based surveillance. Lancet Infect Dis 2015;15(3):301–9.

19. Measles Fact Sheet N286. World Health Organization. 2015. Available at: http://www.who.int/mediacentre/factsheets/fs286/en/. Accessed February 6, 2016.

20. Dayan GH, Rubin S. Mumps outbreaks in vaccinated populations: are available mumps vaccines effective enough to prevent outbreaks? Clin Infect Dis 2008; 47(11):1458.

21. van Loon FP, Holmes SJ, Sirotkin BI, et al. Mumps surveillance–United States, 1988-1993. MMWR CDC Surveill Summ 1995;44(3):1.

22. Reef SE, Plotkin S, Cordero JF, et al. Preparing for elimination of congenital Rubella syndrome (CRS): summary of a workshop on CRS elimination in the United States. Clin Infect Dis 2000;31(1):85.

23. Fleisher G, Henry W, McSorley M, et al. Life-threatening complications of varicella. Am J Dis Child 1981;135(10):896.

24. Hurwitz ES, Barrett MJ, Bregman D, et al. Public health service study on Reye's syndrome and medications. Report of the pilot phase. N Engl J Med 1985; 313(14):849.

25. Vento S, Garofano T, Renzini C, et al. Fulminant hepatitis associated with hepatitis A virus superinfection in patients with chronic hepatitis C. N Engl J Med 1998; 338(5):286.

26. Daniels D, Grytdal S, Wasley A, et al. Surveillance for acute viral hepatitis - United States, 2007. Centers for Disease Control and Prevention (CDC). MMWR Surveill Summ 2009;58(3):1.

27. Bruce MG, Rosenstein NE, Capparella JM, et al. Risk factors for meningococcal disease in college students. JAMA 2001;286(6):688.

28. Centers for Disease Control and Prevention (CDC). Recommendation of the Advisory Committee on Immunization Practices (ACIP) for use of quadrivalent meningococcal conjugate vaccine (MenACWY-D) among children aged 9 through 23 months at increased risk for invasive meningococcal disease. MMWR Morb Mortal Wkly Rep 2011;60(40):1391.

29. Rosenstein NE, Perkins BA, Stephens DS, et al. The changing epidemiology of meningococcal disease in the United States, 1992-1996. J Infect Dis 1999; 180(6):1894.

30. MacNeil JR, Rubin L, Folaranmi T, et al. Use of Serogroup B Meningococcal Vaccines in Adolescents and Young Adults: Recommendations of the Advisory Committee on Immunization Practices, 2015. MMWR Morb Mortal Wkly Rep 2015; 64(41):1171–6.

31. Winer RL, Lee SK, Hughes JP, et al. Genital Human Papillomavirus Infection: Incidence and Risk Factors in a Cohort of Female University Students. Am J Epidemiol 2003;157(3):218–26.

32. CDC. Epidemiology and prevention of vaccine-preventable diseases. 12th edition. Chapter 10: human papillomavirus. Available at: cdc.gov/vaccines/pubs/pinkbook/hpv.html. Accessed February 21, 2016.

33. Woodman CB, Collins SI, Young LS. The natural history of cervical HPV infection: unresolved issues. Nat Rev Cancer 2007;7:11–22.

34. Markowitz LE, Liu G, Hariri S, et al. Prevalence of HPV after introduction of the vaccination program in the United States. Pediatrics 2016;137(3): e20151968.
35. Wong KK, Jain S, Blanton L, et al. Influenza-associated pediatric deaths in the United States, 2004-2012. Pediatrics 2013;132(5):796.
36. Available at: http://www.nvic.org/about/nvic-board-members-staff-and-volunteers. aspx. Accessed February 28, 2016.
37. Offit PA, Quarles J, Gerber MA, et al. Addressing parents' concerns: do multiple vaccines overwhelm or weaken the infant's immune system? Pediatrics 2002; 109(1):124–9.
38. Wakefield AJ, Murch SH, Anthony A, et al. Retraction: Ileal-lymphoid-nodular hyperplasia, non-specific colitis, and pervasive developmental disorder in children [retracted 2010]. Lancet 1998;35(9103):637–41.
39. Deer B. How the case against the MMR vaccine was fixed. BMJ 2011;342: c5347.
40. Hurley AM, Tadrous M, Miller ES. Thimerosal-containing vaccines and autism: a review of recent epidemiologic studies. J Pediatr Pharmacol Ther 2010;15(3): 173–81.
41. Andrews N, Miller E, Grant A, et al. Thimerosal exposure in infants and developmental disorders: a retrospective cohort study in the United Kingdom does not support a causal association. Pediatrics 2004; 114(3):584.
42. Madsen KM, Lauritsen MB, Pedersen CB, et al. Thimerosal and the occurrence of autism: negative ecological evidence from Danish population-based data. Pediatrics 2003;112(3 Pt 1):604.
43. Parker SK, Schwartz B, Todd J, et al. Thimerosal-containing vaccines and autistic spectrum disorder: a critical review of published original data. Pediatrics 2004; 114(3):793.
44. Price CS, Thompson WW, Goodson B, et al. Prenatal and infant exposure to thimerosal from vaccines and immunoglobulins and risk of autism. Pediatrics 2010;126(4):656–64.
45. Nyhan B, Reifler J. Does correcting myths about the flu vaccine work? An experimental evaluation of the effects of corrective information. Vaccine 2015;33(3): 459–64.
46. Liddon NC, Leichliter JS, Markowitz LE. Human papillomavirus vaccine and sexual behavior among adolescent and young women. Am J Prev Med 2012;42: 44–52.
47. CDC. Information for health care professionals about adolescent vaccines. Available at: cdc.gov/vaccines/who/teens/downloads/hcp-factsheet.pdf. Accessed February 28, 2016.
48. Opel DJ, Mangione-Smith R, Robinson JD, et al. The influence of provider communication behaviors on parental vaccine acceptance and visit experience. Am J Public Health 2015;105(10):1998–2004.

Absence Epilepsy
More than a Little Illness

Kelly J. Butler, MPAS, PA-C

KEYWORDS

- Absence epilepsy • Petit mal • EEG • Generalized epilepsy • Ethosuximide
- Childhood epilepsy • Idiopathic epilepsy • 3-Hz spike and wave

KEY POINTS

- Absence seizures are an important condition to accurately and promptly recognize in affected children because failure to do so increases the child's risk of injury and, if untreated, can lead to decline in academic performance.
- Absence seizures are a form of generalized epilepsy that primarily affects children and are characterized by brief episodes of loss of consciousness that typically occur multiple times a day without treatment.
- A diagnosis of absence seizures is made by obtaining a history consistent with the condition and a specific pattern on an electroencephalogram; treatment is with antiseizure medications and patients must be monitored for side effects, efficacy, and development of any new seizure types.

DEFINITIONS
Seizure

A manifestation of disordered brain electrical discharges; a single event, a symptom of cerebral dysfunction (**Box 1**).

The particular characteristics of a seizure episode depend on the area of the brain where the disordered electrical activity occurs and the extent of the involvement (**Fig. 1**).

Epilepsy

A medical condition associated with a tendency toward recurrent seizures without a transient cause.

1. Hyponatremia → seizure
   A provoked seizure, once sodium level returns to normal no further tendency toward seizures, therefore not representative of epilepsy
2. No trigger → seizure + no trigger → seizure
   Two or more unprovoked seizures, high likelihood of recurrence = epilepsy

Disclosure Statement: The author has nothing to disclose.
Comprehensive Epilepsy Program, Children's Health, Children's Medical Center Dallas, 1935 Medical District Drive, Dallas, TX 75235, USA
E-mail address: KELLY.BUTLER@childrens.com

Physician Assist Clin 1 (2016) 627–637
http://dx.doi.org/10.1016/j.cpha.2016.05.008
2405-7991/16/© 2016 Elsevier Inc. All rights reserved.

Box 1
Causes and signs of seizures

Some causes of seizures

- Trauma
- Toxins
- Infection
- Metabolic disturbance
- Underlying brain dysfunction.

Signs of a seizure: changes in sensation, motor control, or consciousness

- Stiffening
- Jerking
- Loss of tone (astatic or atonic)
- Change in sensation (tingling, numbness)
- Autonomic (sweating, pallor, nausea)
- Impaired consciousness

Epilepsy can be expressed in many ways, but individual patients' seizures tend to be stereotypical discrete episodes of symptoms. One patient may always have whole body convulsions, another may always experience sensory changes without impairment of consciousness, whereas yet another patient may have several different seizure types as part of an epilepsy syndrome. Absence seizures are just one possible type of generalized seizures. A patient having recurrent absence seizures has epilepsy and may have an epilepsy syndrome, such as childhood absence epilepsy or juvenile absence epilepsy (**Box 2**).

Absence seizures are often first brought to attention by a child's teacher, who reports that the child sometimes suddenly stops what the child is doing or saying and stares off into space and is unresponsive but then quickly resumes prior activity.

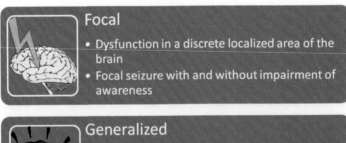

Focal
- Dysfunction in a discrete localized area of the brain
- Focal seizure with and without impairment of awareness

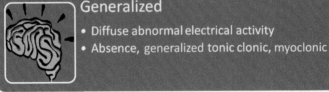

Generalized
- Diffuse abnormal electrical activity
- Absence, generalized tonic clonic, myoclonic

Fig. 1. Characteristics of seizure episode.

Box 2

Childhood absence epilepsy—a generalized epilepsy syndrome

Epilepsy syndrome

- A specific set of signs and symptoms, including features of the epilepsy such as age at onset, seizure types, and electroencephalogram (EEG) findings, that, when occurring together, are known to suggest a certain course of the condition and that guide management.[1]

Petit mal is French for little illness

- It is not just a little illness; children can experience serious consequences if untreated.
- Untreated absence seizures place the child at risk for injury during a seizure as well as of having cognitive difficulties.
- Can lead to psychological problems such as anxiety, low self-esteem, and decreased confidence and motivation.

Parents may report that their child frequently zones out and nothing they can do can interrupts the child's daydream (**Box 3**).

There are many reasons other than epilepsy for a child to temporarily have decreased responsiveness, but these concerns should be followed by further questioning to determine whether the child may be experiencing absence seizures and thus have epilepsy, requiring treatment (**Box 4**).

If the history suggests that episodes are situational or are interruptible, they are less likely to represent seizures and are more consistent with behavioral episodes related to boredom, attention deficit, or daydreaming. If the events are not interruptible but do not occur multiple times daily, last longer than 30 seconds, and are associated with some impairment after resolution, then they may represent seizure activity of a different type (such as focal seizure with impaired consciousness, also known as complex partial seizures) (**Box 5**).

The neurons that are firing abnormally during an absence seizure are those in the pathways that enable people to transition from being awake to being asleep, thus absence seizures manifest in an abrupt impairment of consciousness. The child may freeze in the middle of a movement or suddenly stop talking in the middle of a sentence, the eyes typically remain open and fixed, the child appears to be staring or have a blank look on the face, and the child does not respond to any external stimulation (auditory, visual, or tactile) (**Box 6**).

Childhood Absence Epilepsy

Childhood absence epilepsy is a condition that is classified as an idiopathic or genetic generalized epilepsy. The abnormal electrical activity causing the seizures is

---

Box 3

Typical descriptions of absence seizures by parents, caregivers, and teachers

- Daydreams or zones out a lot
- Stares off into space, as though not there
- Does not hear when called
- Is inattentive, takes a while to respond, or does not respond

> **Box 4**
> **Possible explanations for staring spells**
>
> - Daydreaming
> - Attention deficit/inattention
> - Drowsiness
> - Boredom
> - Absence seizures
> - Complex partial seizures

generalized because of hypersynchrony of neurons. It is currently presumed to have a genetic cause, although clear gene defects that reliably result in childhood absence epilepsy have not been identified.[2] Previously, childhood absence epilepsy was thought to be an idiopathic epilepsy syndrome.[3] Childhood absence epilepsy is one of the most common forms of childhood epilepsy[4] and is an epilepsy syndrome that has a good prognosis if identified and treated. It is important for health care providers, specifically pediatric providers, to be familiar with the evaluation, diagnosis, and management of absence seizures.

Health care providers should be able to recognize the symptoms and accurately diagnose absence seizures because there are serious associated risks, even though the seizures may appear to be less severe than other seizure types. If identified and managed appropriately, treatment is usually effective and the condition has a good prognosis, with most children achieving remission before puberty.[5] However, the cognitive impact as well as the psychological and emotional outcomes may persist beyond seizure remission. Furthermore, some children with absence epilepsy later develop convulsive or other seizure types (**Box 7**).

> **Box 5**
> **Absence and complex partial seizures comparison**
>
> *Absence seizure*
> - Impaired consciousness
> - Lasts 5 to 15 seconds
> - Occurs multiple times daily
> - Immediate return to baseline afterward
> - No warning preceding sudden onset
>
> *Complex partial seizure*
> - Impaired consciousness
> - Lasts 1 to 3 minutes
> - Rarely occurs daily, typically occurs occasionally or infrequently
> - Followed by drowsiness, confusion, or other postictal phenomenon
> - Can be preceded by an aura (abnormal sensation or feeling warning of seizure coming)

Box 6
Comparison of typical absence seizures and atypical absence seizures

Typical absence seizures

- Sudden behavioral arrest
- Loss of awareness
- Unresponsive to stimuli
- Blank facial expression
- Abrupt onset and resolution
- Immediate return to baseline
- Occur multiple times a day

Atypical absence seizures

- May have a more gradual onset
- May be slightly longer in duration
- May have eye blinking, fluttering, or eyebrow twitching
- May have oromotor automatisms (licking lips, chewing movements)
- May have slight loss of tone, mild head nod
- May have urinary incontinence
- May have autonomic symptoms: pallor, sweating, nausea

DIAGNOSIS

The median age of onset is 6 years.[6] In a child between the ages of 4 and 10 years, with normal developmental and cognitive history, a report of multiple daily events described as brief sudden arrest of activity and staring with unresponsiveness followed by return to baseline should raise concern for possible childhood absence epilepsy and prompt further evaluation (**Box 8**).

When the history raises concern for seizures, the evaluation involves obtaining clinical history and a physical examination, including thorough neurologic examination; neurophysiologic testing (electroencephalogram [EEG]); and, depending on the results, perhaps neuroimaging (MRI) and laboratory testing (**Fig. 2**).

The EEG pattern associated with absence seizures must be present to accurately diagnose childhood absence epilepsy. An EEG in childhood absence epilepsy shows generalized 3-Hz spike and slow wave discharges that increase with hyperventilation and may be associated with a clinical change during the EEG recording; the background of the EEG is normal (**Fig. 3**).[6]

Box 7
Risks of uncontrolled seizures

- Injury sustained during a seizure (on playground, at home, bathing, swimming)
- Cognitive decline
- Psychosocial and educational impact
- Absence status epilepticus

Box 8
Typical patients with childhood absence epilepsy

- Healthy children (free of neurologic problems)
- Young, school-aged children (5–10 years old, peak at 6–7 years)
- Girls more often than boys
- Brain is structurally normal
- May be having learning struggles secondary to seizures but not cognitively impaired otherwise

---

If the history is consistent (age at onset of symptoms, child is otherwise neurologically normal, description of events is suggestive of absence seizures) and the EEG shows generalized 3-Hz spike and wave with a normal background and no other epileptiform discharges, then the diagnosis of childhood absence epilepsy should be made[7] If the EEG does not show this pattern then the clinician must consider the other epilepsies associated with absence seizures as well as the other causes of decreased responsiveness, such as complex partial seizures or other nonepileptic causes listed previously.

Hyperventilation is a common trigger for absence seizures in children with untreated absence epilepsy.[6] Even before obtaining an EEG, at the initial consultation, health care providers can use a supervised trial of hyperventilation to attempt to elicit a typical absence seizure to guide the diagnosis. This trial requires a cooperative child giving a consistent, good effort at hyperventilation for 3 to 5 minutes; this can be performed while blowing on a pinwheel. If a typical absence seizure is provoked by this test, then a presumptive diagnosis can be made and treatment started. EEG should still be obtained for confirmation and to rule out risk for other seizure types. Once the diagnosis of childhood absence epilepsy has been made, treatment should be initiated.

Goal of treatment: complete seizure freedom without unwanted side effects of medication

Even 1 brief seizure a week places the child at risk for injury and/or cognitive dysfunction

---

Most patients with childhood absence epilepsy can achieve complete seizure control with adequate doses of medication; therefore, therapy should be adjusted until that goal is achieved. Although a child may have been having dozens of seizures daily at time of diagnosis and a reduction to a couple of seizures per week after starting treatment is a dramatic improvement, the therapy should be adjusted until no seizures are observed. The treatment does not cure the epilepsy, but it controls the manifestation of the condition; it suppresses seizure activity. Medication adherence is very important and the therapy must be taken consistently because the tendency for seizure recurrence remains.

The subtle nature of absence seizures may lead to unrecognized seizures and the outward appearance of complete seizure control when the child may still be experiencing seizures. In the clinic setting, performing hyperventilation during follow-up visits can help providers gauge whether seizures are adequately controlled. If hyperventilation in the clinical setting provokes an absence seizure, the child is not adequately treated and medication adjustments should be considered. Any persistent seizures present risks and indicate suboptimal seizure control. The presence of

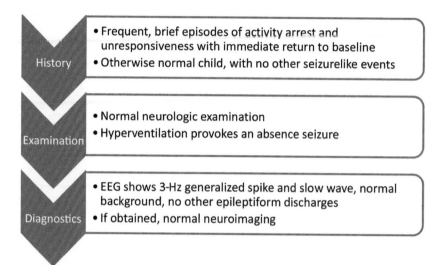

Fig. 2. Diagnosis evaluation.

ongoing or recurrent academic struggles may indicate that seizures are not adequately controlled.

MEDICATIONS

Treatment options for absence seizures include ethosuximide, valproic acid, and lamotrigine. For childhood absence epilepsy, ethosuximide is the drug of choice and should be considered first line in children having only absence seizures and no other findings on EEG except those expected with childhood absence epilepsy.[8] It works by increasing seizure threshold, suppressing spike and slow wave activity, and depressing nerve transmission in the cortex.

> Drug of choice for childhood absence epilepsy: ethosuximide.

The medication should be started at a low dose and gradually titrated to an effective and tolerated dose.

> Start low, go slow

There is an established therapeutic trough serum drug level; this is the amount of medication that usually controls seizures without adverse side effects. In children, this is weight dependent because medications are dosed in milligrams per kilogram per day, typically given in 2 to 3 divided doses. The medication is usually started at 10 mg/kg/d divided twice a day and titrated by 5 to 10 mg/kg/d every 7 days until the desired response is achieved. The typical therapeutic dose is 20 to 30 mg/kg/ d divided twice a day (can be as low as 15 mg/kg/d or up to 40 mg/kg/d). The maximum daily dose is 60 mg/kg/d or 2000 mg daily, whichever is less. Blood tests

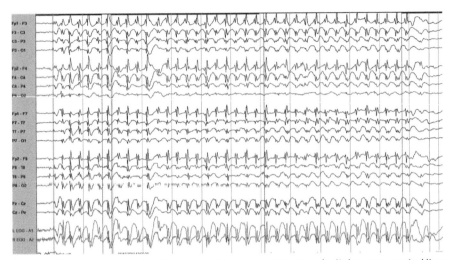

Fig. 3. An EEG showing classic 3-Hz spike and slow wave. Between the light green vertical lines equals 1 second, and there are 3 spikes followed by a slow wave within each second. There are generalized discharges throughout the leads and bilaterally (blue is left and red is right).

can also evaluate serum levels to further guide dosing to achieve optimum seizure control without unwanted side effects. Typical therapeutic ethosuximide trough level is between 40 and 100 μg/mL. The medication is available as a liquid suspension and in gel capsules. It generally is well tolerated. Common side effects are gastrointestinal distress (abdominal pain, nausea, vomiting, diarrhea, anorexia, weight loss), drowsiness, and sleep disturbances. These side effects usually either improve with time or can be managed by adjusting how and when the medication is given. If gastrointestinal symptoms are bothersome, giving the medication with food and administering the medication in capsule formulation often improves tolerability. Less common but serious side effects include blood disorders, skin rash (Stevens-Johnson syndrome), and drug-induced lupus.

Caution

Be aware that ethosuximide, although very effective for absence seizures, does not control other seizure types. Patients who are also experiencing other seizures types, such as generalized tonic-clonic seizures, will not be successfully treated with ethosuximide monotherapy. Ethosuximide may be used as an adjunctive therapy to treat the absence seizures, but another medication is necessary to treat other seizure types.

Once the therapy is started and the initial goal dose is reached, clinicians can expect to achieve complete seizure control within 4 to 16 weeks.[8] If there are still seizures at that time, then the dose should be gradually advanced every few weeks until the seizures are controlled, the maximum dose has been reached (based on milligrams per kilogram per day or by serum level), or the patient cannot tolerate increased doses. If the child continues to have seizures despite maximal safe or tolerable dose, then another medication, such as valproic acid or lamotrigine, should be considered. If the medication is discontinued because of intolerability or allergy it is important to notate that as the reason. A medication failure caused by lack of efficacy is a negative prognostic indicator, compared with a medication discontinued because of allergy or side effects. If the seizures are not readily controlled with the second medication, then a pediatric neurologist or epileptologist should be consulted (**Box 9**).

Phenytoin and phenobarbital are ineffective in treating absence seizures. There are also some medications to avoid because of the potential for worsening generalized epilepsies, including absence seizures: carbamazepine, vigabatrin, gabapentin, tiagabine.[7]

After complete seizure control has been attained, the therapy should be continued for at least 2 to 3 years. Even in the case of adequate seizure control, during this time the dose may need to be increased to adjust for growth as the child gains weight. Once it has been 2 years since the last seizure (or the first-time hyperventilation did not provoke an absence seizure in clinic if seizures were not observed by parents/teachers), the patient should be reevaluated to determine the likelihood that the patient has outgrown the tendency for recurrent seizures. The history should be reviewed to assess for risk factors for seizure recurrence and a repeat EEG should be considered, especially if there has been concern that there may be unrecognized seizures. If the EEG is normal, the risks of a trial off medication should be reviewed so that a decision can be made regarding whether to wean off the medication.

If it is decided to trial off medical therapy, then the medication should be gradually weaned over several weeks. Even in the best-case scenario of a patient who quickly achieved complete seizure control once starting therapy, has not had a seizure in 2 years on monotherapy with the first medication tried, and has a normal EEG, there is a risk of seizure recurrence with the taper off the antiseizure medication. However, if the seizures recur, the patient usually becomes seizure free again once the medication is restarted. The highest risk of seizure recurrence is in the first 6 to 12 months off medication. Children of driving age should be cautioned to avoid driving (or participating in any high-risk activities) for 6 months after they have been weaned off their antiseizure medication (**Box 10**).

DIFFERENTIAL DIAGNOSIS

The presence of absence seizures does not necessarily indicate childhood absence epilepsy. Although this is the most common childhood epilepsy associated with absence seizures, it is not the only epilepsy syndrome that can manifest with absence seizures. If a child has absence seizures but also other seizure types, by definition that is not childhood absence epilepsy. Furthermore, onset of absence seizures in older children (>10 years of age) usually is not suggestive of childhood absence epilepsy. These children frequently also have a history of generalized tonic-clonic seizures and myoclonic seizures. Some adults may have absence seizures. A history of absence seizures along with generalized tonic-clonic seizures that started in a slightly older child suggests the syndrome of juvenile absence

---

Box 9
Medications for childhood absence epilepsy

- Ethosuximide
- Valproic acid
- Lamotrigine

> **Box 10**
> **Risk factors for seizure recurrence in childhood absence epilepsy after stopping medication because of being seizure free for more than 2 years**
>
> - Family history of epilepsy
> - History of absence status epilepticus
> - Recent abnormal EEG
> - Seizures did not come under control quickly with the start of therapy
> - Seizures required 2 or more medications to remain under control

epilepsy. Similarly, an older age of onset but with myoclonic seizures as well as absence and generalized tonic-clonic seizures is suggestive of juvenile myoclonic epilepsy (**Table 1**).

Note that adolescents who are experiencing myoclonic seizures sometimes do not realize that the jerks they are having are abnormal and therefore they do not report them, and their parents may not have seen them because they often occur in the early morning. This history can be elicited with direct questioning by describing the lightninglike jerks of the upper body that tend to occur in the early morning or on awakening. Likewise, parents may think their child's episodes of decreased responsiveness are normal childhood behavior and present with a history of convulsions or jerking episodes but not mention episodes of decreased responsiveness until specifically asked about them. Obtaining an accurate and thorough history is very important in evaluating any paroxysmal episode (**Fig. 4**).

Table 1
Epilepsy syndromes associated with absence seizures

	CAE	Juvenile Absence Epilepsy	Juvenile Myoclonic Epilepsy	Epilepsy with Myoclonic Absences
Typical Age of Onset (y)	5–9	9–13	Adolescence	1–12
Male/Female Ratio	Girls > boys	Girls > boys	Girls = boys	Boys > girls
Seizure Types	Absences: very frequent	Absence: less frequent, commonly have GTC seizures	GTC, myoclonic, and absence: less common, less frequent, less impairment, and briefer than in CAE	Frequent daily absences with myoclonic jerking of upper body, arms, or legs; most patients also have GTCs and atonic (drop) seizures
Prognosis	Good, likely to outgrow	Moderate, unlikely to outgrow, may continue to have GTCs in adulthood	Moderate, do not outgrow, do well as long as treatment is continued	Poor, difficult to treat, most develop learning disability, rarely outgrow

Abbreviations: CAE, childhood absence epilepsy; GTC, generalized tonic-clonic.

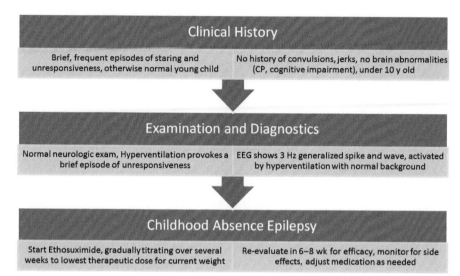

Fig. 4. Evaluating absence epilepsy.

SUMMARY

Childhood absence epilepsy is a common childhood form of epilepsy with a good prognosis. However, because of the subtle nature of the absence seizures associated with the condition, it may go unrecognized and thus untreated. There is significant morbidity associated with untreated absence seizures because they place the child at risk for injury and cognitive dysfunction. Learning the signs of absence seizures, how to evaluate a child for possible absence epilepsy, and how to initiate treatment are important to all health care providers who care for children.

REFERENCES

1. International League Against Epilepsy, EPILEPSY SYNDROMES. Available at: https://www.epilepsydiagnosis.org/syndrome/epilepsy-syndrome-groupoverview.html. Accessed February 26, 2016.
2. Berg AT, Berkovic SF, Brodie MJ, et al. Revised terminology and concepts for organization of seizures and epilepsies: report of the ILAE Commission on Classification and Terminology, 2005-2009. Epilepsia 2010;51:676.
3. Proposal for revised classification of epilepsies and epileptic syndromes. Commission on Classification and Terminology of the International League Against Epilepsy. Epilepsia 1989;30:389.
4. Berg AT, Shinnar S, Levy SR, et al. How well can epilepsy syndromes be identified at diagnosis? A reassessment 2 years after initial diagnosis. Epilepsia 2000;41:1269.
5. Callenbach PM, Bouma PA, Geerts AT, et al. Long-term outcome of typical childhood absence epilepsy: Dutch Study of Epilepsy in Childhood. Epilepsy Res 2009;83:249.
6. Sadleir LG, Farrell K, Smith S, et al. Electroclinical features of absence seizures in childhood absence epilepsy. Neurology 2006;67:413.
7. Medina M, Bureau M, Hirsch E, et al. Childhood absence epilepsy. In: Bureau M, Genton P, Dravet C, et al, editors. Epileptic syndromes in infancy, childhood and adolescence. 5th edition. England: John Libbey Eurotext; 2012. p. 277.
8. Glauser TA, Cnaan A, Shinnar S, et al. Ethosuximide, valproic acid, and lamotrigine in childhood absence epilepsy. N Engl J Med 2010;362:790.

Urinary Tract Infections in the Pediatric Patient

Meredith E. Alley, PA

KEYWORDS

- Urinary tract infection • Cystitis • Pyelonephritis • Urologic anatomic abnormality
- Vesicoureteral reflux • Voiding dysfunction

KEY POINTS

- Appropriate collection of a urine specimen is paramount to diagnosing a urinary tract infection (UTI). A urine culture in a pre–potty trained child should be a catheterized sample or suprapubic aspirate.
- Obtaining a clear history of symptoms is helpful in determining whether the UTI is likely to be cystitis or pyelonephritis, which then informs type and duration of treatment.
- Current recommendations and clinical acumen should be used to determine which patients should have radiologic imaging after a UTI.
- Differentiating between anatomic abnormalities versus suboptimal habits as the cause of UTIs is essential to correctly treating the underlying cause of the UTI.
- Medical and surgical management options to treat the underlying cause of UTIs are reviewed as well as review of medical options to prevent UTIs.

INTRODUCTION

Urinary tract infections (UTIs) in the pediatric patient are common. One study estimates that UTIs affect 2.4% to 2.8% of children each year.[1] Three common times for UTIs are infancy,[2] potty training age,[3] and when a female patient becomes sexually active.[4] Appropriate diagnosis and treatment is essential to protecting renal health. Determining whether further workup is needed after a UTI occurs is important. UTIs can be related to voiding and stooling behaviors,[3] but can also have an underlying anatomic abnormality as the cause[5]; determining the underlying cause is paramount to helping prevent future UTIs.

PATHOGENESIS

Although bacterial pathogens are the most common cause of UTIs, fungal, parasitic, and viral UTIs can also occur but are much less frequent.[6] UTIs caused by bacteria have 3 main origins: retrograde ascent from enteral bacteria colonizing urethral and

The author has nothing to disclose.
Division of Urology, Children's Hospital of Philadelphia, 34th Street and Civic Center Boulevard, Richard D. Wood Building, 3rd Floor, Philadelphia, PA 19104, USA
E-mail address: alleym@email.chop.edu

Physician Assist Clin 1 (2016) 639–660
http://dx.doi.org/10.1016/j.cpha.2016.06.002
2405-7991/16/$ – see front matter © 2016 Elsevier Inc. All rights reserved.

vaginal tissue, nosocomial caused by catheterization, and hematogenous spread through systemic infection. The most common origin is retrograde ascent.[7] *Escherichia coli*, *Klebsiella*, *Proteus*, *Enterococcus*, *Citrobacter*, *Serratia*, and *Pseudomonas* were found to be the most common urinary pathogens in several recent pediatric studies, with *E coli* being the most common causative bacteria.[8,9] Any child can get a UTI; however, there are certain risk factors and congenital anomalies that can increase a child's risk.

ANATOMIC ABNORMALITY RISK FACTORS FOR URINARY TRACT INFECTIONS

Anatomic abnormalities that may increase the risk of a UTI include vesicoureteral reflux (VUR), ureterocele, ectopic ureter, megaureter, ureterovesical junction obstruction, multicystic dysplastic kidney, ureteropelvic junction obstruction (UPJO), horseshoe kidney, cross-fused renal ectopia, kidney stones, posterior urethral valves (PUV), neurogenic bladder, bladder diverticulum, bladder duplication, urogenital sinus, and cloaca. VUR is the most common underlying congenital abnormality that is found in the workup of febrile UTIs; the other less common congenital causes that are risk factors for UTI are often diagnosed based on antenatal imaging findings that are confirmed postnatally.

Congenital ureteral abnormalities that can increase the risk of a UTI include VUR, ureterocele, ectopic ureteral insertion, and megaureter. VUR increases the risk of a kidney infection by giving bacteria in the bladder easier access to the kidney. VUR is a congenital abnormality where the ureter does not tunnel correctly into the bladder and, therefore, urine washes back up from the bladder toward the kidney. VUR is diagnosed with either a voiding cystourethrogram or contrast-enhanced ultrasonography (see section on Imaging in Urinary Tract Infections), and is graded from low grade (grade 1) to high grade (grade 5; **Fig. 1**).[10]

Another ureteral anomaly that can increase the risk of a UTI is a ureterocele, a balloonlike out pouching at the end of the ureter, which is an abnormality in ureteral formation. The ureterocele can cause urine to not drain normally, cause bladder outlet obstruction by obstructing the bladder neck if the ureterocele is large, and can be associated with VUR and thus increase the risk of a UTI.[10] An ectopic ureter is a ureter that inserts into an abnormal location; common insertion sites of an ectopic ureter include the urethra, vagina, and bladder neck. The abnormal insertion site is associated commonly with slowed urinary drainage along with an increased risk of VUR, thus increasing the risk of UTI (**Figs. 2–4**).[10]

Megaureter is an abnormally dilated ureter; this occurs owing to a segment of ureter near the ureterovesical junction that does not have normal peristalsis; if there is sluggish drainage or inadequate drainage such as with a ureterovesical junction obstruction or if there is associated VUR, there is an increased risk of UTI.[10]

Renal abnormalities that can increase the risk of UTI are multicystic dysplastic kidney, UPJO, horseshoe kidney and cross-fused renal ectopia. Multicystic dysplastic kidney is a congenital anomaly that is composed of a collection of cysts and nonfunctioning renal parenchyma.[10] When a multicystic dysplastic kidney is present, there is an increased risk of contralateral VUR, which increases the risk of UTI (**Fig. 5**).[11]

UPJO occurs when there is a narrowed segment of ureter where the ureter inserts into the renal pelvis or when there is an extrinsic compression of the UPJ by a crossing vessel. UPJO causes the kidney to not drain well and can increase the risk of UTI (**Fig. 6**).[10]

A horseshoe kidney, where the kidneys are joined by an isthmus of tissue and their ascent is stopped by the inferior mesenteric artery, carries an increased risk of VUR and UTI (**Fig. 7**).[12]

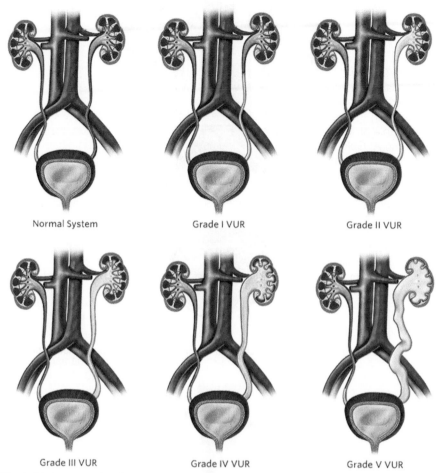

Normal System   Grade I VUR   Grade II VUR

Grade III VUR   Grade IV VUR   Grade V VUR

Fig. 1. Vesicoureteral reflux. (*Courtesy of* The Children's Hospital of Philadelphia, Philadelphia, PA.)

Cross-fused renal ectopia usually occurs when one of the kidneys is attached to the lower pole of the other kidney and is on the side opposite that it normally is. Cross-fused kidneys have an increased risk of VUR and thus UTI.[13] Another renal-level risk factor for UTIs is genitourinary stones. Stones can serve as a nidus for infection and if the stone persists, it can cause recurrent UTIs.[14]

Bladder and urethral anomalies that can predispose to UTI are PUV, neurogenic bladder, bladder diverticulum, bladder duplication, urogenital sinus, and cloaca. PUV is a congenital abnormality where a valve leaflet is present in the posterior urethra, causes lower urinary tract obstruction and hydronephrosis (dilation in the urinary tract), and increases the risk of UTIs because of an increased incidence of VUR, hydronephrosis, and incomplete bladder emptying (**Figs. 8** and **9**).[10]

Neurogenic bladder increases the risk of UTI because the bladder does not contract and empty normally. If there is a large postvoid residual, there can be stagnant urine where bacteria can multiply and cause a UTI. Common causes of neurogenic bladder in the pediatric population include spina bifida, tethered spinal cord, and spinal cord

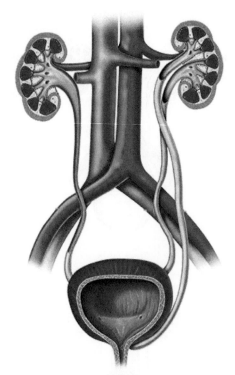

Fig. 2. Ectopic ureter. (*Courtesy of* The Children's Hospital of Philadelphia, Philadelphia, PA.)

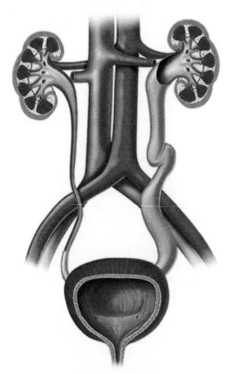

Fig. 3. Megaureter. (*Courtesy of* The Children's Hospital of Philadelphia, Philadelphia, PA.)

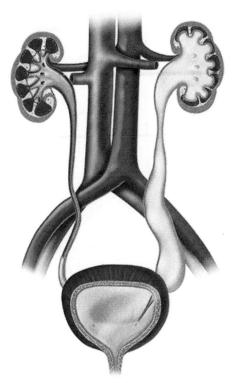

Fig. 4. Ureterovesical junction obstruction. (*Courtesy of* The Children's Hospital of Philadelphia, Philadelphia, PA.)

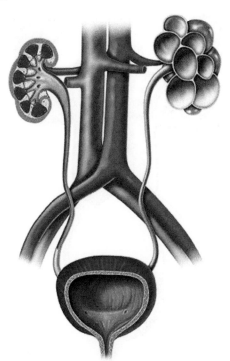

Fig. 5. Multicystic dysplastic kidney. (*Courtesy of* The Children's Hospital of Philadelphia, Philadelphia, PA.)

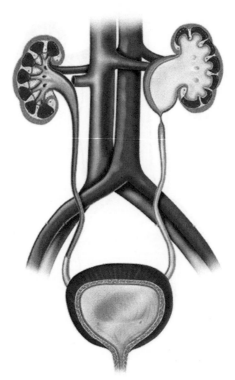

Fig. 6. Ureteropelvic junction obstruction. (*Courtesy of* The Children's Hospital of Philadelphia, Philadelphia, PA.)

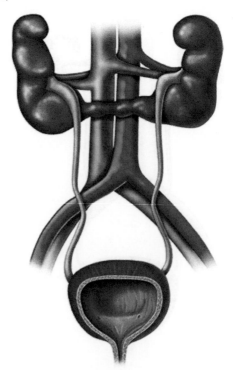

Fig. 7. Horseshoe kidney. (*Courtesy of* The Children's Hospital of Philadelphia, Philadelphia, PA.)

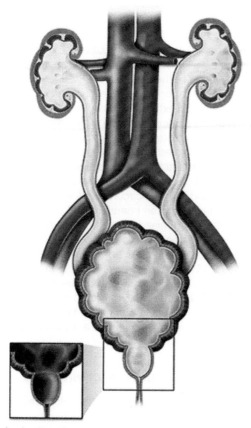

Fig. 8. Posterior urethral valves. (*Courtesy of* The Children's Hospital of Philadelphia, Philadelphia, PA.)

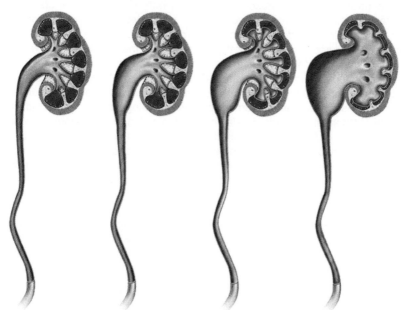

Fig. 9. Hydronephrosis. (*Courtesy of* The Children's Hospital of Philadelphia, Philadelphia, PA.)

injury.[10] Congenital or acquired bladder diverticulum are outpouchings of the bladder, a weakening in the bladder wall. Bladder diverticulum can make it difficult to empty the bladder well and thereby increase the risk of UTI.[10] Bladder duplication, although rare, can increase the risk of UTI by causing incomplete emptying of the bladder.[10] Urogenital sinus, where there is a single external opening for the urethra and vagina, can increase the risk of a UTI owing to increased associated incidence of spinal anomalies, hydrometrocolpos, and bladder distention.[10] Cloaca increases the risk of UTI because there is a single opening for the urethra, vagina, and anus, and this can result in poor drainage of the urinary system and because there is an increased risk of VUR.[15]

Risk factors for UTI other than anatomic anomalies include age, status of the immune system, female sex, and being uncircumcised. In the first 6 months of life, there is an increased risk of UTI owing to an immature and developing immune system.[16] Diabetes and an immunocompromised state are also risk factors for UTI.[7] Some research has shown that being uncircumcised increases an infant's risk for a UTI until 1 year of age. One study reported that the incidence of UTI in an uncircumcised male in the first year of life was 2.15%, whereas it was 0.22% in circumcised males.[17] It is thought that the foreskin can be colonized with bacteria, which in turn can increase the risk of retrograde urethral ascension.[2,18] After 1 year of age, females are more likely to have a UTI than males. This is thought to be owing to the proximity of the anus to the urethra and likelihood of bacteria that are colonizing the perineum gaining access to the urethra.[5]

BEHAVIORAL RISK FACTORS FOR URINARY TRACT INFECTIONS

In addition to anatomic abnormality risk factors, behavioral factors and habits can increase the risk of developing a UTI. Holding of the urine can create stagnant urine, which can give bacteria a chance to multiply, stick to the bladder wall and ultimately cause a UTI.[6,19] Dysfunctional voiding is the discoordination of the normal voiding process of contraction of the detrusor muscle along with relaxation of the bladder neck and external sphincter. Infrequent voiding and incomplete emptying are considered types of dysfunctional voiding. Dysfunctional voiding increases the risk of a UTI.[6,19–21]

Constipation is another risk factor that can increase the likelihood of developing a UTI.[22] The definition of what constitutes constipation is varied, but some indicators can be large stools, painful stools, and infrequent stools, which is defined by some as less than once daily and by others as fewer than 3 bowel movements a week.[23,24] Constipation can be from an organic pathologic cause, but is most often functional.[22] Often times children delay defecation owing to the memory of a painful bowel movement or busyness with another activity.[22] Withholding of stool can result in further constipation and start an unpleasant cycle of constipation.[22] A child who is constipated is often not able to fully relax his pelvic floor muscles to fully empty the bladder when he voids, leaving a postvoid residual.[24] It is also hypothesized that constipation can cause overgrowth of uropathogens by changing the gastrointestinal flora and thus increases the risk of a UTI.[24–26]

Suboptimal water intake is thought to be a risk factor for UTIs, although no large studies have documented this. Inadequate water intake is thought to be a risk factor for UTI because the kidneys and bladder will not be flushed as often as they should be and results in stagnant urine. Suboptimal water intake is also a risk factor for constipation, which in turn increases risk of UTI.

Potty training can be a high-risk time for UTIs.[3] The child is learning when and how to contract and relax their pelvic floor muscles and how to empty their bladder. Children who are potty training often forget to void and need reminders to void on a timed schedule. Constipation can often occur during potty training because the child is learning to hold their stool, which further increases the risk of a UTI during this time. Any child is at higher risk of UTI during potty training, but especially children with anatomic abnormalities of the genitourinary tract. A vibrating watch, which can be set for intervals several hours apart, can act as an external reminder to void routinely and can assist with adhering to timed voiding recommendations.

Finally, the onset of sexual activity increases the risk of a UTI in females by the introducing bacteria into the urethra.[4]

SYMPTOMS OF URINARY TRACT INFECTIONS
Symptoms by Age

Infants can have a more atypical presentation, including vomiting, feeding intolerance, diarrhea, lethargy, and fever of unknown origin.[8,9] Fever of an unknown origin is the most common presenting symptom in infants. One study stratified the risk of febrile UTIs based on age of the infant: in females 0 to 3 months of age, the risk was 7.5%; from 3 to 6 months of age, 5.7%; from 6 to 12 months of age, 8.3%; and greater than 12 months of age, 2.1%. In febrile males less than 3 months of age, the investigators found the incidence of febrile UTI to be 2.4% in circumcised males and 20.1% in uncircumcised males.[27]

Factors that have been shown to increase the likelihood that a febrile female infant will have a UTI are white race, temperature of 39°C or higher, fever for more than 2 days, and no known cause for fever.[28,29] For febrile males, factors that increase the likelihood of UTI include nonblack race, fever for more than 24 hours, uncircumcised status, temperature of greater than 39°C, and no other source of fever.[30,31] In a febrile infant, being uncircumcised should increase clinical suspicion for a UTI.

Young children with a UTI often have presenting symptoms of dysuria, gross hematuria, urgency, frequency, fever, urinary incontinence, difficulty voiding, nausea, vomiting, lethargy, oliguria, polyuria, abdominal pain, and flank pain.[8] Fever is the most common symptom in the pre–potty trained child. A high fever typically indicates that the UTI is pyelonephritis. A low-grade temperature can accompany an episode of cystitis.[31] Adolescents with cystitis can have the lower urinary symptoms as listed. Flank pain, nausea, vomiting, and high fever often occur with pyelonephritis.[8] Symptoms usually start as lower urinary symptoms and then progress to symptoms associated with pyelonephritis if left untreated. This is consistent with ascending infection. In some patients, flank pain and fever are the first recognizable symptoms. Sexually transmitted infections (STIs) should be in the differential diagnosis of an adolescent female who presents with urinary symptoms. Some studies have shown that if vaginal discharge is present, there is a decreased likelihood that it is a UTI and an increased likelihood that it is an STI, whereas other studies show that the diagnosis of UTI cannot be precluded even if vaginal discharge is present, if urinary symptoms are present. Other studies show that UTI and STI may occur at the same time owing to the common risk factor of sexual activity and recommend that any adolescent female presenting with urinary symptoms should be tested for both UTI and STI.[32] Testing for STIs in this population presenting with urinary complaints should be considered.[32,33]

INITIAL WORKUP AND ACUTE TREATMENT FOR URINARY TRACT INFECTIONS

Urine should be sent for microscopic urinalysis to look for nitrites, leukocyte esterase, and white blood cells. Urinalysis showing nitrites and leukocyte esterase is suspicious for a UTI.[8] Certain bacteria are more likely to produce nitrites than others. E coli,

Klebsiella, and *Proteus* can produce nitrites; *Enterococcus* does not. If nitrites are positive there is increased specificity for a UTI, but if negative, this does not rule out a UTI. If the urine has not been in the bladder long enough for the bacteria to convert nitrate to nitrite, the nitrite may be falsely negative. Pyuria and bacteriuria are suspicious for a UTI.[8]

Urine culture is the gold standard and essential to diagnosing and appropriately treating a UTI. Urine should always be sent for culture and sensitivities, before starting antibiotic treatment.[34] Even 1 dose of antibiotic before obtaining a urine sample can result in sterilization of the urine.

In the pre–potty trained child, a urine specimen should be collected via urethral catheterization or suprapubic aspiration (SPA).[8] This is the most accurate way to obtain a urine sample.[35] Sterile catheterization seems to be more routinely performed over SPA, likely owing to provider experience and comfort with performing urethral catheterization versus SPA. SPA is considered more invasive than catheterization and often requires ultrasound guidance to be performed successfully. Times when SPA may be deemed necessary are when tight phimosis or significant labial adhesions are present, precluding urethral catheterization.

Although it is often tempting to collect a bagged specimen to avoid having to catheterize a child, it is not reliable enough and the risk of a contaminated specimen is too high.[35] A bagged specimen is more likely to be contaminated with skin flora, especially in an uncircumcised male. If a bagged specimen is obtained, the urine is dipped and negative for indicators of infection, and the child is not significantly ill, monitoring is an option. If the bagged specimen urine is suspicious for a UTI, a catheterized or SPA specimen should be obtained and sent for urine culture.[8,36] A bagged specimen can be helpful if negative but cannot be interpreted accurately if positive. If the child is potty trained and able to give a clean catch midstream specimen, this can be sent for culture rather than obtaining a catheterized or SPA urine sample.[37]

There is controversy over what quantity of colony-forming units (CFU) truly constitutes a UTI. One approach is that a CFU greater than 100,000 is necessary to diagnose a UTI from a voided specimen, a CFU of greater than 50,000 from a catheterized specimen, and any growth from an SPA specimen.[8] Another approach is that a colony count of greater than 50,000 by any collection method is considered sufficient for diagnosis of a UTI.[35] These CFU are a suggested count but are not absolute. If the colony count is low and a patient is symptomatic, recollection or treatment should be considered in light of the clinical scenario. A specimen growing many different organisms is most likely a contaminated specimen and recollection should be considered. The urine should be dipped in the office; if it is suspicious for a UTI and the patient is symptomatic, empiric antibiotic treatment should be started.

Empiric treatment should be based on age, prior urine cultures and sensitivities, and local antibiotic sensitivity patterns and then tailored to the final culture sensitivities.[8,38] Cephalexin (Keflex), sulfamethoxazole-trimethoprim (Bactrim), and amoxicillin and clavulanic acid (Augmentin) are often considered for first-line oral treatment.[35] Nitrofurantoin should not be considered for patients with high fevers or who are systemically ill because it does not have good tissue penetration.[39] Patients with a normal urinary system and an uncomplicated course of cystitis can receive a 2- to 4-day course of antibiotic treatment.[8,40] If there is an anatomic abnormality, longer treatment should be considered. Pyelonephritis requires a longer course of treatment.

Treatment also varies depending on the age of the child. An infant under 2 months of age should undergo a catheterized urine culture or suprapubic aspirate as part of the evaluation for fever of unknown origin or sepsis. It is recommended that a febrile infant less than 28 days of age receive a septic workup, empiric antibiotics, and admission to the hospital owing to the risk of serious bacterial infection.[41] UTIs are the most common cause of serious bacterial infection in infants younger than 3 months of age.[41] Infants, 1 to 3 months of age with a fever of an unknown origin should have a urinalysis and urine culture; admission and intravenous (IV) antibiotic versus oral treatment should be based on the appearance of the child, and clinician and family comfort and preference. The 2011 American Academy of Pediatrics guidelines estimate that the incidence of UTI in a febrile infant from 2 to 24 months of age is approximately 5%.[27] If no source for the fever can be identified in this age group, the urine should be checked.[8,35,42]

In infants 2 to 24 months of age, treatment of febrile UTIs should be for 7 to 14 days.[8] In this group, oral and parenteral treatment show the same efficacy unless the child is too ill to tolerate oral treatment.[43] Infants older than 2 months of age can often be treated at home with oral antibiotic therapy.[8] If they have a high fever that is nonresponsive to antipyretics, are unable to tolerate fluids, or are systemically not doing well and appear toxic, treatment with intramuscular antibiotics, IV antibiotics, and/or admission to the hospital should be considered.[8]

If a patient is not responding to appropriate antibiotic treatment after 48 to 72 hours, consider imaging of the kidneys to rule out a renal abscess.[8,35] If a child or adolescent is having significant dysuria, phenazopyridine (Pyridium) can be considered as an adjunct to antibiotics for symptomatic relief.

Prompt treatment of UTIs to prevent ascending infection, pyelonephritis, renal abscess, renal scarring, and urosepsis is important. Urosepsis occurs when the urinary pathogen becomes blood borne and causes bacteremia. Urosepsis can be life threatening. UTI in the setting of a kidney stone should be promptly treated because a stone can become obstructing and an infection in an obstructed system is a risk factor for urosepsis.[44]

A patient can be asymptomatic but found to have bacteria in the bladder, often found on routine urine screening. This is referred to as bacteriuria or bacterial colonization. This can occur in any patient but occurs at an increased rate in patients on clean intermittent catheterization or who have an indwelling foreign object such as a ureteral stent or suprapubic tube.[45] Routine screening for asymptomatic bacteriuria in a healthy child is not recommended. Treatment of asymptomatic bacteriuria is usually deferred owing to potential risk of antibiotic treatment and potential development of a resistant organism. Patients undergoing an invasive urologic surgical procedure should have a preoperative urine culture and preoperative antibiotic treatment owing to the risk of bacteremia and sepsis. A preoperative urine culture can guide appropriate perioperative antibiotic coverage. Further study is needed to determine the exact urologic surgeries that require a preoperative urine culture.[46]

FOLLOW-UP EVALUATION OF INITIAL AND RECURRENT URINARY TRACT INFECTIONS WITH IMAGING

Routine workup of a febrile UTI in a pediatric patient should include a renal bladder ultrasound (RBUS).[35] Imaging a few weeks after the UTI is thought to be preferred if the child is clinically improving with antibiotic therapy; E coli endotoxin can potentially cause dilation of the ureter and kidney during the infection, which may then resolve a few weeks after the UTI.[35] RBUS can assess for size of the kidneys, scarring to the kidneys, cysts, hydronephrosis, stones, bladder wall thickening, trabeculated bladder, distended bladder, and postvoid residual.[47,48] Findings on RBUS that are suspicious for VUR are urothelial thickening and dilation of the ureter and kidney. A normal RBUS does not exclude the presence of VUR as patients with VUR often have a normal

RBUS.[48] Any patient with a febrile UTI and an abnormal RBUS most likely warrants further workup with a voiding cystourethrogram (VCUG) to assess for VUR. Although RBUS is a noninvasive way to assess the kidneys and bladder, it is not a sensitive test for renal scarring.[49]

If the RBUS is abnormal in an infant with a first febrile UTI, or if there is a recurrent febrile UTI even with a normal RBUS, further imaging with a VCUG should be considered.[8] A VCUG is done under fluoroscopy and involves insertion of a catheter into the bladder, injection of a contrast solution to fill and cycle the bladder, and monitoring for VUR with pulse fluoroscopy during the filling and voiding phases. The American Academy of Pediatrics guidelines published in 2011 recommend that, in patients from 2 to 24 months of age who have an initial febrile UTI, "a VCUG is not recommended routinely after the first UTI" if the RBUS is normal.[35] The guidelines do acknowledge that "this guideline does not indicate an exclusive course of treatment or serve as a standard of care."[35] The American Academy of Pediatrics guideline is helpful in considering what the appropriate workup of a patient with a febrile UTI should be, but should not replace seeing the entire clinical scenario that encompasses a patient, exercising good clinical judgment, and providing individualized care. When to obtain a VCUG after a febrile UTI remains a subject of debate. If there is more than 1 febrile UTI, an abnormal RBUS, or the patient is younger than 2 months of age, the general consensus is to obtain a VCUG.

A diagnostic imaging option that is offered at some pediatric institutions that can be used in place of a VCUG is contrast-enhanced ultrasonography. It is performed in ultrasound and involves a catheter that is inserted into the bladder, a solution composed of microbubbles flows through the catheter and fills the bladder, the bladder cycles, and the bladder, ureters, and kidneys are imaged by ultrasound to see if any of the bubbles can be seen in the ureters or kidneys, which would indicate VUR. The advantage of this study versus a traditional VCUG is that there is no radiation involved in the test. Although the radiation involved in a traditional VCUG is low, being able to avoid radiation entirely with contrast-enhanced ultrasonography is an advantage.[50,51]

If there is significant dilation of the kidney and/or ureter and no VUR is present on VCUG, a functional study such as a MAG-3 Renal scan or MRI Urogram may be indicated to see how well the kidney is functioning and how well it is draining. Surgical intervention may be needed to help the kidney drain better and preserve the function it has. A MAG-3 renal scan is performed in nuclear medicine and involves a catheter in the bladder to ensure the bladder is completely empty and an IV through which a tracer (technetium 99m-mercaptoacetyl triglycine) is injected. Imaging of the kidneys and bladder is obtained in nuclear medicine to determine how quickly the kidneys take up the tracer to determine the functional split of the kidneys and then furosemide (Lasix) is given to determine how quickly the kidneys wash the tracer out.[10]

MR urogram provides both functional and anatomic data. An MR urogram involves a catheter in the bladder, injection of gadolinium through an IV, and then MRI to assess the kidneys, ureters, and bladder. Three-dimensional imaging is then reconstructed to reflect the anatomy. Many calculations are done to determine kidney function as well as the washout of the kidneys to determine if there is an obstruction. The benefit of the MR urogram over the MAG3 Renal Scan is that it does not involve radiation and gives more detailed anatomic information such as being able to identify ectopic ureteral insertion or a crossing vessel at the UPJ.[52]

In a patient with febrile UTIs, a dimercaptosuccinic acid (DMSA) renal scan can assess functional split of the kidneys and renal defects. A DMSA scan involves IV injection of the tracer and then subsequent imaging of the kidneys in nuclear medicine to look at the uptake of the tracer by the kidneys. An area of the kidney that does not enhance demonstrates injury to the kidney. Renal defects can represent either an acute insult to the kidney if there has been a recent episode of pyelonephritis, represent renal scarring if there is a history of febrile UTIs, or it may represent renal dysplasia, a congenital abnormal formation of the kidneys that can often be associated with high-grade VUR. Kidneys that have numerous wedgelike defects bilaterally are often referred to as having a Swiss cheese appearance.[53] One approach to imaging patients with febrile UTIs is referred to as the "top-down" approach. This involves imaging the kidneys with a DMSA scan before obtaining a VCUG. If the ultrasound and DMSA scan are negative, a VCUG is often not obtained because there are no renal defects seen. If the DMSA is positive, a VCUG is often then obtained to assess for VUR as a potential cause of the renal defects.[49] The "bottom-up" approach is the more conventional approach to imaging children with febrile UTIs: obtaining a VCUG first to assess for VUR and then, if positive, considering DMSA to assess for renal defects. There does not seem to be consensus about which is the better approach; there are benefits and drawbacks to each approach, including a catheter with VCUG, IV, with DMSA, radiation associated with both, and potentially missing VUR in patients where DMSA is negative and VCUG is not obtained.

SERUM LABORATORY EVALUATION IN RECURRENT URINARY TRACT INFECTIONS

If there are recurrent febrile UTI's and evidence of renal scarring on RBUS or DMSA, particularly bilaterally, obtaining a serum creatinine level is prudent to assess for overall impact on renal function.[54,55] An estimated glomerular filtration rate can then be calculated based on the serum creatinine and patient height. If the creatinine is elevated or estimated glomerular filtration rate is decreased, consultation with a pediatric nephrologist is warranted to assess for chronic kidney disease (CKD) and renal insufficiency.[54] Nephrologists assess staging and progression of CKD, monitor serum creatinine and blood pressure and assess for proteinuria. Urology typically manages the underlying cause of the recurrent UTIs and nephrology typically follows and manages renal insufficiency.

Procalcitonin is a marker in the blood that may be ordered at the time of concern for pyelonephritis; it has increased sensitivity compared with C-reactive protein and white blood cell count as an indicator of active pyelonephritis and may be a predictor of renal scarring.[56]

FUNCTIONAL TESTING

A uroflow can be obtained to assess a child's voiding. The child voids, ideally with a full bladder, into the uroflow, a container that catches and then analyzes the flow rate. The flow pattern is a reflection of pelvic floor musculature. It captures peak flow, staccato voiding, dampened flow rate, and urgency. This can help to identify patients who have dysfunctional voiding and who are not relaxing their pelvic floor muscles fully when they void (**Figs. 10–12**).[21]

After voiding in the toilet or in the uroflow, a patient's bladder can be scanned with a handheld ultrasound device to determine to what degree they are able to empty their bladder. A large postvoid residual is a risk factor for UTI.[6,20]

TREATMENT AND PREVENTION OF RECURRENT URINARY TRACT INFECTIONS

Treatment of recurrent UTIs should address the underlying cause of the UTI and should include methods aimed at prevention of further UTI's. Preventative methods include addressing bowel and bladder dysfunction, antibiotic prophylaxis, cranberry

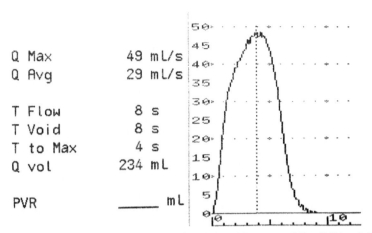

Fig. 10. Relaxed bell-shaped flow pattern with urgency. (*Courtesy of* The Children's Hospital of Philadelphia, Philadelphia, PA.)

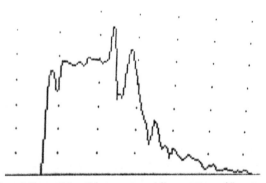

Fig. 11. Overall relaxed flow with mild staccato voiding pattern. (*Courtesy of* The Children's Hospital of Philadelphia, Philadelphia, PA.)

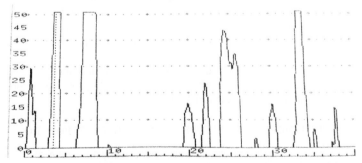

Fig. 12. Significant staccato voiding pattern on uroflow. (*Courtesy of* The Children's Hospital of Philadelphia, Philadelphia, PA.)

extract, D-mannose, probiotics, and surgical correction of VUR or underlying anatomic cause of UTI.

Medical Treatment

If the VCUG does show VUR, antibiotic prophylaxis should be considered, especially in infants and patients with higher grades of VUR. When to use antibiotic prophylaxis is a subject of ongoing debate. The RIVUR (Randomized Intervention for Children With Vesicoureteral Reflux) study included children with grades 1 to 4 VUR and showed that the risk of febrile or symptomatic UTIs was reduced by one-half in the patients on antibiotic prophylaxis versus placebo.[57] It reported no difference in renal scarring between the groups.[57] It did show that patients with grade 3 to 4 VUR were more likely to have a febrile or symptomatic recurrence than patients with grade 1 to 2 VUR.[57] It reported that patients with VUR and bowel and bladder dysfunction showed particular benefit to being on antibiotic prophylaxis.[57] The thought process behind antibiotic prophylaxis is that, if you are able to keep the urine that is in the bladder sterile through a low dose of antibiotic, even if the urine refluxes, if it does not have bacteria in it, then it is not an increased risk factor for pyelonephritis. Antibiotic prophylaxis can decrease the likelihood of pyelonephritis, but does not work absolutely because you can get bacteria that are resistant to the antibiotic agent that was selected for prophylaxis, a breakthrough UTI. A study in Australia showed that antibiotic prophylaxis did decrease modestly the risk of UTI in patients with VUR or recurrent UTI.[58] This study did not assess whether antibiotic prophylaxis decreased risk of renal scarring.[58]

A once daily low-dose antibiotic can be considered to try to help break a cycle of recurrent UTIs, even in patients without an anatomic abnormality. One study showed that antibiotic prophylaxis modestly decreases the risk of UTIs in children with recurrent UTIs.[58] It is thought that the irritative voiding symptoms of a UTI can produce holding behaviors owing to the memory of pain associated with voiding. It is thought that a UTI makes the bladder more susceptible to a UTI soon after having one, most common in the subsequent 6 months. Often prophylaxis is continued for a period of 6 months and then discontinued.[58] This can be done in conjunction with working on voiding and stooling habits and water drinking to try to decrease the risk factors for recurring UTIs.

If a patient has recurrent UTIs that are caused by *E coli*, a cranberry extract supplement may aid in preventing further *E coli* UTIs. The cranberry extract supplement mimics the *E coli* fimbriae binding site, *E coli* are more likely to bind to the cranberry extract than the bladder wall, helping to prevent a UTI. Studies have shown varying results as to the efficacy of cranberry juice or cranberry supplements in preventing *E coli* UTIs.[7,59,60] D-Mannose is thought to potentially decrease the risk of certain types of UTIs by blocking the adherence factors of certain types of bacteria. Further clinical study is needed.[61] Probiotics are thought to potentially reduce the risk of UTIs by altering the vaginal and intestinal flora to reduce uropathogens. Further clinical studies are needed for further recommendations.[62]

Behavioral and Bowel and Bladder Dysfunction Treatment

It is generally recommended that, once potty trained, children void every 2 to 3 hours on average to give the bladder a chance to empty and void out any bacteria that are inside. Keeping track of voiding habits on voiding diaries can be helpful.[3] Using a stool under the feet of a child can be helpful if their feet do not touch the floor. This helps their pelvic floor muscles to relax more fully when they void and defecate. Ensuring they bring their pants and underpants down to their ankles will help them to relax to void. Sitting to void versus standing can further help to relax the pelvic floor.[19,63]

The goal is to take away constipation as a risk factor. The definition of constipation is not uniformly agreed upon, but softer, more frequent bowel movements are what are focused on. Increased dietary fiber and increased water intake often can be helpful.[64,65] Polyethylene glycol (Miralax) can be used to help achieve softer, more frequent bowel movements.[66] Referral to a gastroenterologist may be necessary if constipation does not resolve with these measures. Taking advantage of the gastrocolic reflex, sitting to attempt to stool soon after a meal can be helpful in achieving a daily bowel movement.[22] Reviewing the Bristol Stool Scale or Rome Criteria with a patient can be helpful in identifying constipation; keeping stooling diaries can be helpful in determining frequency of stools.[19,22,67,68]

If a uroflow demonstrates that a child is not relaxing their pelvic floor muscles to void or the postvoid bladder scan shows a large postvoid residual, biofeedback can be initiated. Biofeedback involves electromyogram electrodes being placed on the perineum of the patient; these electrodes transmit their muscle contraction and relaxation onto a screen where they can visualize the activity of their pelvic floor muscles. Biofeedback teaches the child how to isolate the pelvic floor muscles to contract and relax them appropriately to fully relax to void and to empty their bladder completely. Often, several sessions of biofeedback are necessary to learn pelvic floor relaxation. Studies have shown that biofeedback can help to decrease the risk of developing a UTI and help to decrease VUR by treating the underlying voiding dysfunction.[69]

Meeting with a behavioral psychologist or a psychologist who specializes in urology can be helpful for discussing motivational techniques, understanding barriers to adhering to behavioral modification recommendations such as timed voiding and water drinking, and thereby optimizing patient outcomes.[70]

Surgical treatment

A variety of surgical procedures may be considered, depending on the cause of the recurrent UTIs. If recurrent febrile UTIs occur despite antibiotic prophylaxis and treatment of bowel and bladder dysfunction in a patient with high-grade VUR, surgical treatment of VUR should be considered.[9,49] This treatment includes ureteral reimplantation and endoscopic treatments. Ureteral reimplantation is a surgery where the ureter is tunneled further into the bladder at a nonrefluxing angle. Ureteral reimplantation can be done through an open procedure or through a minimally invasive laparoscopic/robotic approach.[49] An endoscopic treatment approach is where a bulking substance, hyaluronic acid/dextranomer (Deflux), can be injected into the ureteral orifice to provide antireflux backing of the ureter.[49] Ureteral reimplantation is a more definitive surgical approach to repair VUR.

Other surgical treatments of UTIs may include the following.

- If recurrent febrile UTIs occur in a male infant, especially one who has an anatomic urologic abnormality, circumcision should be considered.[71]
- A cystoscope can be used to incise a ureterocele. Future ureteral reimplantation may be needed to correct any associated VUR that may occur with the ureterocele.[10]
- Patients with ectopic ureters may undergo ureteral reimplantation, marsupialization of the ureter into bladder, end cutaneous ureterostomy, upper pole partial nephroureterectomy, or ureteroureterostomy.[10]
- Ureteral reimplantation is the definitive treatment for an obstruction at the ureterovesical junction or for a highly refluxing megaureter.[72] Pyeloplasty is the primary method for addressing UPJO. The narrowed segment of ureter is excised and then the remaining ureter is reattached to the pelvis of the kidney.[10] Stones can serve as a nidus for infection[7] and can often be large, staghorn calculi. Entire

removal of the stone is often best achieved through percutaneous nephrolithotomy.[73]

- Cystoscopy and incision of PUV is the primary method of surgical management of PUV. Incision of the valves does not eliminate the risk of UTI in a patient with PUV as they often have persistent risk factors including VUR, and incomplete bladder emptying, but incision will decrease the risk by resolving the obstructive element. Neurogenic bladders have abnormal innervation, do not contract normally, and often do not empty completely, predisposing to UTI.[6] Clean intermittent catheterization is often instituted to help empty the bladder.[6] If the pressure in a bladder is high at low filling volumes and UTIs recur, bladder augmentation or vesicostomy are other surgical options to help decompress the bladder and prevent UTIs.[10]

LONG-TERM CONCERNS WITH RECURRENT URINARY TRACT INFECTIONS
Recurrent Afebrile Urinary Tract Infections

Recurrent afebrile UTIs are not associated with long-term renal damage. Prompt treatment is recommended to prevent ascending infection and pyelonephritis. However, repeat exposure to antibiotic treatment can be associated with resistance to antibiotics and increased risk of *Clostridium dificile*.[74] Lost time from school and parental time away from work is an incurred cost.[7] Monetary costs associated with repeat visits to the health care provider's office and associated treatment should be considered.[5]

Recurrent Febrile Urinary Tract Infections

Recurrent febrile UTIs and subsequent renal damage can increase the long-term risk of developing hypertension. The exact incidence of hypertension in children with renal scarring owing to febrile UTIs is unknown, but is estimated to occur in 17% to 30% of children with significant renal scarring.[75] Renal scarring after pyelonephritis ranged from 26% to 49% in 1 metaanalytic study and was estimated to be 30% in another study.[75,76] Annual screening of blood pressure for hypertension and urinalysis for proteinuria is recommended in a patient with a history of VUR and renal damage (**Figs. 13 and 14**).[55]

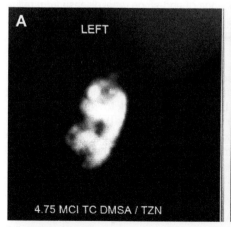 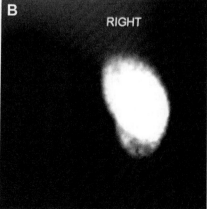

Fig. 13. Dimercaptosuccinic acid with renal defects. (*A*) Multiple renal defects. (*B*) Normal appearing kidney. (*Courtesy of* The Children's Hospital of Philadelphia, Philadelphia, PA.)

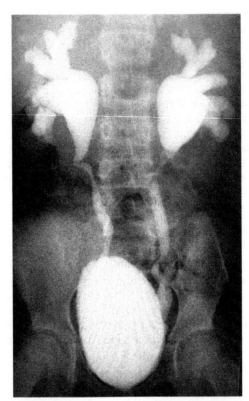

Fig. 14. Voiding cystourethrogram showing bilateral high grade vesicoureteral reflux. (*Courtesy of* The Children's Hospital of Philadelphia, Philadelphia, PA.)

Recurrent febrile UTIs can cause scarring to the kidneys and result in renal insufficiency. The prevention of recurrent febrile UTIs is focused on protecting renal reserve. One study estimates that reflux nephropathy is the cause of 19% of end-stage renal disease in children worldwide, and is lower in the United States.[77] One study reported a slower progression to end-stage renal disease in patients with VUR as the cause of CKD versus other underlying causes of CKD.[54] The exact incidence of end-stage renal disease from reflux nephropathy and recurrent pyelonephritis is unknown, but all efforts should be made to prevent recurrent febrile UTIs, renal scarring and chronic renal insufficiency.

Future Research

Correctly diagnosing, treating, and subsequently working up a patient with a UTI is important to identifying underlying risk factors for UTIs and preventing recurrent afebrile and febrile UTIs. Recurrent febrile UTIs increase the risk for renal scarring, hypertension, and renal insufficiency. Further research to elucidate genetic factors associated with recurrent UTIs and with renal scarring could be helpful in determining who is at greatest risk for UTI and for renal scarring. Focusing on preventative therapies for this subset of patients could potentially help prevent CKD.

REFERENCES

1. Freedman AL, Urologic Diseases in America Project. Urologic diseases in North America Project: trends in resource utilization for urinary tract infections in children. J Urol 2005;173:949–54.

2. Zorc JJ, Levine DA, Platt SL, et al. Clinical and demographic factors associated with urinary tract infection in young febrile infants. Pediatrics 2005;116:644–8.
3. Wan J, Kaplinsky R, Greenfield S. Toilet habits of children evaluated for urinary tract infection. J Urol 1995;154:797–9.
4. Vincent CR, Thomas TL, Reyes L, et al. Symptoms and risk factors associated with first urinary tract infection in college age women: a prospective cohort study. J Urol 2013;189:904–10.
5. Foxman B. Epidemiology of urinary tract infections: incidence, morbidity, and economic costs. Am J Med 2002;113(Suppl 1A):5S–13S.
6. Chang SL, Shortliffe LD. Pediatric urinary tract infections. Pediatr Clin North Am 2006;53:379–400, vi.
7. Ma JF, Shortliffe LM. Urinary tract infection in children: etiology and epidemiology. Urol Clin North Am 2004;31:517–26, ix–x.
8. Robinson JL, Finlay JC, Lang ME, et al, Canadian Paediatric Society, Infectious Diseases and Immunization Committee, Community Paediatrics Committee. Urinary tract infections in infants and children: diagnosis and management. Paediatr Child Health 2014;19:315–25.
9. Bell LE, Mattoo TK. Update on childhood urinary tract infection and vesicoureteral reflux. Semin Nephrol 2009;29:349–59.
10. Wein AJ, Kavoussi LR, Campbell MF. Campbell-Walsh urology. In: Wein AJ, Kavoussi LR, Partin AW, et al, editors. 10th edition. Philadelphia: Elsevier Saunders; 2012.
11. Flack CE, Bellinger MF. The multicystic dysplastic kidney and contralateral vesicoureteral reflux: protection of the solitary kidney. J Urol 1993;150:1873–4.
12. Cascio S, Sweeney B, Granata C, et al. Vesicoureteral reflux and ureteropelvic junction obstruction in children with horseshoe kidney: treatment and outcome. J Urol 2002;167:2566–8.
13. Guarino N, Tadini B, Camardi P, et al. The incidence of associated urological abnormalities in children with renal ectopia. J Urol 2004;172:1757–9 [discussion: 1759].
14. Bichler KH, Eipper E, Naber K, et al. Urinary infection stones. Int J Antimicrob Agents 2002;19:488–98.
15. Warne SA, Wilcox DT, Ledermann SE, et al. Renal outcome in patients with cloaca. J Urol 2002;167:2548–51 [discussion: 2551].
16. James-Ellison MY, Roberts R, Verrier-Jones K, et al. Mucosal immunity in the urinary tract: changes in sIgA, FSC and total IgA with age and in urinary tract infection. Clin Nephrol 1997;48:69–78.
17. Schoen EJ, Colby CJ, Ray GT. Newborn circumcision decreases incidence and costs of urinary tract infections during the first year of life. Pediatrics 2000;105:789–93.
18. To T, Agha M, Dick PT, et al. Cohort study on circumcision of newborn boys and subsequent risk of urinary-tract infection. Lancet 1998;352:1813–6.
19. van Gool JD, Hjalmas K, Tamminen-Mobius T, et al. Historical clues to the complex of dysfunctional voiding, urinary tract infection and vesicoureteral reflux. The International Reflux Study in Children. J Urol 1992;148:1699–702.
20. Chandra M. Reflux nephropathy, urinary tract infection, and voiding disorders. Curr Opin Pediatr 1995;7:164–70.
21. Vesna Z, Milica L, Marina V, et al. Correlation between uroflowmetry parameters and treatment outcome in children with dysfunctional voiding. J Pediatr Urol 2010;6:396–402.

22. Baker SS, Liptak GS, Colletti RB, et al. Constipation in infants and children: evaluation and treatment. A medical position statement of the North American Society for Pediatric Gastroenterology and Nutrition. J Pediatr Gastroenterol Nutr 1999; 29:612–26.

23. Fontana M, Bianchi C, Cataldo F, et al. Bowel frequency in healthy children. Acta Paediatr Scand 1989;78:682–4.

24. Giramonti KM, Kogan BA, Agboola OO, et al. The association of constipation with childhood urinary tract infections. J Pediatr Urol 2005;1:273–8.

25. Combs AJ, Van Batavia JP, Chan J, et al. Dysfunctional elimination syndromes–how closely linked are constipation and encopresis with specific lower urinary tract conditions? J Urol 2013;190:1015–20.

26. Neumann PZ, DeDomenico IJ, Nogrady MB. Constipation and urinary tract infection. Pediatrics 1973;52:241–5.

27. Shaikh N, Morone NE, Bost JE, et al. Prevalence of urinary tract infection in childhood: a meta-analysis. Pediatr Infect Dis J 2008;27:302–8.

28. Ishimine P. The evolving approach to the young child who has fever and no obvious source. Emerg Med Clin North Am 2007;25:1087–115, vii.

29. Gorelick MH, Shaw KN. Clinical decision rule to identify febrile young girls at risk for urinary tract infection. Arch Pediatr Adolesc Med 2000;154:386–90.

30. Finnell SM, Carroll AE, Downs SM. Subcommittee on Urinary Tract I. Technical report: diagnosis and management of an initial UTI in febrile infants and young children. Pediatrics 2011;128:e749–70.

31. Shaikh N, Morone NE, Lopez J, et al. Does this child have a urinary tract infection? JAMA 2007;298:2895–904.

32. Huppert JS, Biro F, Lan D, et al. Urinary symptoms in adolescent females: STI or UTI? J Adolesc Health 2007;40:418–24.

33. Shapiro T, Dalton M, Hammock J, et al. The prevalence of urinary tract infections and sexually transmitted disease in women with symptoms of a simple urinary tract infection stratified by low colony count criteria. Acad Emerg Med 2005;12:38–44.

34. Whiting P, Westwood M, Watt I, et al. Rapid tests and urine sampling techniques for the diagnosis of urinary tract infection (UTI) in children under five years: a systematic review. BMC Pediatr 2005;5:4.

35. Subcommittee on Urinary Tract Infection, Steering Committee on Quality Improvement and Management, Roberts KB. Urinary tract infection: clinical practice guideline for the diagnosis and management of the initial UTI in febrile infants and children 2 to 24 months. Pediatrics 2011;128:595–610.

36. McGillivray D, Mok E, Mulrooney E, et al. A head-to-head comparison: "clean-void" bag versus catheter urinalysis in the diagnosis of urinary tract infection in young children. J Pediatr 2005;147:451–6.

37. Vaillancourt S, McGillivray D, Zhang X, et al. To clean or not to clean: effect on contamination rates in midstream urine collections in toilet-trained children. Pediatrics 2007;119:e1288–93.

38. Edlin RS, Shapiro DJ, Hersh AL, et al. Antibiotic resistance patterns of outpatient pediatric urinary tract infections. J Urol 2013;190:222–7.

39. Ramlakhan S, Singh V, Stone J, et al. Clinical options for the treatment of urinary tract infections in children. Clin Med Insights Pediatr 2014;8:31–7.

40. National Collaborating Centre for Women's and Children's Health (UK). Urinary tract infection in children: diagnosis, treatment and long-term management. London: RCOG Press 2013; 2007.

41. Hamilton JL, John SP. Evaluation of fever in infants and young children. Am Fam Physician 2013;87:254–60.
42. Newman TB. The new American Academy of Pediatrics urinary tract infection guideline. Pediatrics 2011;128:572–5.
43. Hodson EM, Willis NS, Craig JC. Antibiotics for acute pyelonephritis in children. Cochrane Database Syst Rev 2007;(4):CD003772.
44. Wagenlehner FM, Lichtenstern C, Rolfes C, et al. Diagnosis and management for urosepsis. Int J Urol 2013;20:963–70.
45. Nicolle LE. Asymptomatic bacteriuria. Curr Opin Infect Dis 2014;27:90–6.
46. Nicolle LE. Asymptomatic bacteriuria: when to screen and when to treat. Infect Dis Clin North Am 2003;17:367–94.
47. Giorgi LJ Jr, Bratslavsky G, Kogan BA. Febrile urinary tract infections in infants: renal ultrasound remains necessary. J Urol 2005;173:568–70.
48. Wallace SS, Zhang W, Mahmood NF, et al. Renal ultrasound for infants younger than 2 months with a febrile urinary tract infection. AJR Am J Roentgenol 2015; 205:894–8.
49. Koyle MA, Shifrin D. Issues in febrile urinary tract infection management. Pediatr Clin North Am 2012;59:909–22.
50. Berrocal T, Gaya F, Arjonilla A, et al. Vesicoureteral reflux: diagnosis and grading with echo-enhanced cystosonography versus voiding cystourethrography. Radiology 2001;221:359–65.
51. Darge K, Troeger J. Vesicoureteral reflux grading in contrast-enhanced voiding urosonography. Eur J Radiol 2002;43:122–8.
52. Dickerson EC, Dillman JR, Smith EA, et al. Pediatric MR urography: indications, techniques, and approach to review. Radiographics 2015;35:1208–30.
53. Goldraich NP, Goldraich IH. Update on dimercaptosuccinic acid renal scanning in children with urinary tract infection. Pediatr Nephrol 1995;9:221–6 [discussion: 227].
54. Novak TE, Mathews R, Martz K, et al. Progression of chronic kidney disease in children with vesicoureteral reflux: the North American Pediatric Renal Trials Collaborative Studies Database. J Urol 2009;182:1678–81.
55. Peters CA, Skoog SJ, Arant BS Jr, et al. Summary of the AUA guideline on management of primary vesicoureteral reflux in children. J Urol 2010;184:1134–44.
56. Leroy S, Fernandez-Lopez A, Nikfar R, et al. Association of procalcitonin with acute pyelonephritis and renal scars in pediatric UTI. Pediatrics 2013;131: 870–9.
57. Investigators RT, Hoberman A, Greenfield SP, et al. Antimicrobial prophylaxis for children with vesicoureteral reflux. N Engl J Med 2014;370:2367–76.
58. Craig JC, Simpson JM, Williams GJ, et al. Antibiotic prophylaxis and recurrent urinary tract infection in children. N Engl J Med 2009;361:1748–59.
59. Afshar K, Stothers L, Scott H, et al. Cranberry juice for the prevention of pediatric urinary tract infection: a randomized controlled trial. J Urol 2012;188:1584–7.
60. Jepson RG, Craig JC. Cranberries for preventing urinary tract infections. Cochrane Database Syst Rev 2008;(23):CD001321.
61. Altarac S, Papes D. Use of D-mannose in prophylaxis of recurrent urinary tract infections (UTIs) in women. BJU Int 2014;113:9–10.
62. Schwenger EM, Tejani AM, Loewen PS. Probiotics for preventing urinary tract infections in adults and children. Cochrane Database Syst Rev 2015;(12):CD008772.
63. Hellerstein S, Linebarger JS. Voiding dysfunction in pediatric patients. Clin Pediatr (Phila) 2003;42:43–9.

64. Maffei HV, Vicentini AP. Prospective evaluation of dietary treatment in childhood constipation: high dietary fiber and wheat bran intake are associated with constipation amelioration. J Pediatr Gastroenterol Nutr 2011;52:55–9.

65. Nurko S, Zimmerman LA. Evaluation and treatment of constipation in children and adolescents. Am Fam Physician 2014;90:82–90.

66. Candy D, Belsey J. Macrogol (polyethylene glycol) laxatives in children with functional constipation and faecal impaction: a systematic review. Arch Dis Child 2009;94:156–60.

67. Lane MM, Czyzewski DI, Chumpitazi BP, et al. Reliability and validity of a modified Bristol Stool Form Scale for children. J Pediatr 2011;159:437–41.e1.

68. Primavera G, Amoroso B, Barresi A, et al. Clinical utility of Rome criteria managing functional gastrointestinal disorders in pediatric primary care. Pediatrics 2010;125:e155–61.

69. Khen-Dunlop N, Van Egroo A, Bouteiller C, et al. Biofeedback therapy in the treatment of bladder overactivity, vesico-ureteral reflux and urinary tract infection. J Pediatr Urol 2006;2:424–9.

70. Schulman SL, Quinn CK, Plachter N, et al. Comprehensive management of dysfunctional voiding. Pediatrics 1999;103:E31.

71. Singh-Grewal D, Macdessi J, Craig J. Circumcision for the prevention of urinary tract infection in boys: a systematic review of randomised trials and observational studies. Arch Dis Child 2005;90:853–8.

72. Hodges SJ, Werle D, McLorie G, et al. Megaureter. ScientificWorldJournal 2010; 10:603–12.

73. Preminger GM, Assimos DG, Lingeman JE, et al. Chapter 1: AUA guideline on management of staghorn calculi: diagnosis and treatment recommendations. J Urol 2005;173:1991–2000.

74. Levy DG, Stergachis A, McFarland LV, et al. Antibiotics and Clostridium difficile diarrhea in the ambulatory care setting. Clin Ther 2000;22:91–102.

75. Faust WC, Diaz M, Pohl HG. Incidence of post-pyelonephritic renal scarring: a meta-analysis of the dimercapto-succinic acid literature. J Urol 2009;181:290–7 [discussion: 297–8].

76. Hewitt IK, Zucchetta P, Rigon L, et al. Early treatment of acute pyelonephritis in children fails to reduce renal scarring: data from the Italian Renal Infection Study Trials. Pediatrics 2008;122:486–90.

77. Craig JC, Irwig LM, Knight JF, et al. Does treatment of vesicoureteric reflux in childhood prevent end-stage renal disease attributable to reflux nephropathy? Pediatrics 2000;105:1236–41.

Atopic Dermatitis–A New Dawn

Anne Weissler, MMS, PA-C

KEYWORDS

- Atopic dermatitis • Eczema • Topical steroids • Calcineurin inhibitors • *FLG*
- Filaggrin • Th2 • Dupilumab

KEY POINTS

- Atopic dermatitis (AD) results from both abnormalities in the skin, barrier including filaggrin defects, and in the immune system, involving a type 2 T-helper cell response with elevations of interleukin (IL)-4, IL-13, and other cytokines.
- Initial treatment of AD includes moisturization with baths and emollients, bland skin care, application of the appropriate topical steroid, addition of a topical calcineurin inhibitor if needed, and consideration of microbes, mimics, and comorbidities.
- Future systemic treatments may target immune abnormalities that contribute to AD, including dupilumab, an anti-IL-4.

INTRODUCTION

It may not kill you, but it can ruin your life. This phrase is used frequently in the office to describe the morbidity of uncontrolled atopic dermatitis (AD), including pruritus causing loss of sleep, school absence, and other declines in activities of daily living. AD is the most common chronic skin disease in children.[1] Early identification and successful treatment may limit the extent of the disease. The American Academy of Dermatology published updated clinical guidelines for AD but admits gaps in research.[2] The last medications approved for AD were Elidel (December 2001) and Protopic (December 2000).[3] Other medications include topical and oral steroids. Limited options have made treatment frustrating. Fortunately, there are clinical trials for both topical and systemic therapies in progress. Thought leaders have dubbed it a new dawn for AD. Information gathered as a result of this research may transform the understanding and treatment of the disease.

DEFINITION, PREVALENCE, AND RISK FACTORS

AD is characterized as a chronic inflammatory skin condition featuring pruritic, erythematous, scaly papules, vesicles, and plaques that may wax and wane or persist

Conflicts of Interest: The author has no relevant conflicts of interest.
Division of Dermatology, Department of Pediatrics, Cardinal Glennon Children's Hospital, Saint Louis University, 1465 South Grand, St Louis, MO 63104, USA
E-mail address: aweissl@slu.edu

Physician Assist Clin 1 (2016) 661–682
http://dx.doi.org/10.1016/j.cpha.2016.06.004
2405-7991/16/© 2016 Elsevier Inc. All rights reserved.

as chronic lichenified lesions. The word eczema is often used interchangeably with AD. Eczema, however, is a more general term referring to allergic contact dermatitis (ACD), seborrheic dermatitis, psoriasis, AD, and/or other similar conditions. AD is a more specific diagnosis.

AD is often the first presentation of allergic disease. The word atopic refers to a tendency to produce immunoglobulin E (IgE) antibodies after exposure to common substances in the environment such as pollen, house dust mite, and food allergens.[4] Although not every person with AD has an elevated IgE, almost all do. The atopic march describes the sequential development of AD, sensitization to allergens, and finally, progression to asthma and allergic rhinitis.[4] Approximately one-third of patients with AD develop asthma and two-thirds develop allergic rhinitis.[5,6]

Most children with AD develop the condition before entering kindergarten: 45% during the first 6 months of life, 60% during the first year, and 85% before the age of 5.[7] The prevalence of the disease varies according to the study and region. AD affects up to 18% of children and up to 5% of adults.[8] A report from the Centers for Disease Control and Prevention analyzing the National Health Interview Survey found an increase in prevalence of eczema among US children ages 0 to 17 from 7.4% in 1997 to 12.5% in 2011. Analysis of worldwide data suggests that a plateau of around 20% may have been reached in countries with the highest prevalence. It is possible that there are a finite number of individuals susceptible to the condition.[9]

Two strong risk factors for the development of AD include a genetic defect in the filaggrin (FLG) gene (see later discussion) and family history of atopic disease.[10] If 1 parent has AD, asthma, or allergies, there is a 50% chance that the child will have 1 or more of the diseases. If both parents are atopic, the chance is even greater.[7]

Additional risk factors for the development of AD include a higher level of family education, a smaller family size, and residence in an urban environment.[11] These risk factors lead to the hygiene hypothesis. The hypothesis states that a lack of exposure to a variety of microbes may increase the prevalence of AD. Exposure to endotoxins, helminthes, farm animals, dogs, unpasteurized milk, and early day care may be protective against AD.[12]

PATHOGENESIS AND POTENTIAL BIOMARKERS

Although there are no unique biomarkers that help distinguish AD from other conditions, current research gives additional insight into the genetic, immunologic, and environmental influences that contribute to the disease. A review of these concepts gives context to current and future treatment modalities.

There are 2 theories to explain the cause of AD. One is the outside-in hypothesis which states that defects in the epidermal skin barrier allow for increased transepidermal water loss (xerosis) and increased penetration of allergens and microbes, causing an immune reaction. The other is the inside-out hypothesis in which immune defects cause the skin barrier dysfunction. More than likely, these theories are not exclusive. Both play a role in the pathogenesis of AD.[13]

The epidermis of the skin is made of several layers and acts as a barrier to help minimize water loss and protect the body from foreign substances, including microbes and allergens. In 2006, McLean and colleagues[14] demonstrated that the FLG gene has a pivotal role in skin barrier function and in the development of AD. This gene is responsible for the development of the profilaggrin protein. This protein, found in the granular layer of the epidermis, is broken down into smaller FLG molecules.[15] FLG brings structural proteins together, flattening and strengthening the cells to create a strong barrier or matrix.[15,16] This matrix with attached proteins and lipids forms the stratum corneum, the outmost layer of the epidermis.[15] The stratum corneum provides a barrier to prevent penetration of microbes and allergens, and minimize transepidermal water loss. In addition, in the stratum corneum, *FLG* degrades into amino acids and becomes part of the skin's natural moisturizing factor, maintaining hydration of the skin and contributing to the acidic pH.[16,14]

Mutations in the *FLG* gene are common, especially among white patients. Approximately 10% of individuals of European ancestry are heterozygous carriers of a loss-of-function mutation in *FLG*. This results in a 50% reduction in the expression of the protein.[17] An *FLG* gene defect leads to a poorly formed stratum corneum prone to xerosis. The defective skin barrier is at risk for penetration of microbes and allergens causing immune responses.[14] The prevalence of *FLG* mutations in patients with AD is between 20% and 50%. When the *FLG* gene defect is present, the disease is more severe and persistent. It is also more likely to be associated with asthma, peanut allergy, contact dermatitis, and infections such as the herpes virus.[18,19] There are no therapies specifically directed at the gene activity, but this is an obvious area of interest for researchers.

Because not everyone with AD has the *FLG* defect and not everyone with the defect develops AD, it remains just 1 variable. There are several other skin barrier defects, including, but not limited to, a reduction in tight junctions, a deficiency in toll-like receptors, and an increase in thymic stromal lymphopoietin receptors on Langerhans cells. When there are defects in the first few layers of the epidermis, innate immune responses are triggered, beginning the cycle of inflammation.[8,18]

In addition to barrier dysfunction, the inside-out hypothesis argues that immune defects contribute to AD. Patients with the disease have increased type 2 helper T (Th) cells: interleukin (IL)-4, IL-5, IL-13, IL-31, Th17 (IL-17), and Th22 (IL-22) cytokines. These cytokines may decrease the expression of *FLG* and other molecules found in the skin barrier. Lesional and nonlesional skin have abnormalities. When mice are genetically engineered to overexpress Th2 cytokines (IL-4, IL -13, IL-31), they develop skin barrier defects and AD spontaneously.[18] Many of these cytokines are targets for new therapies being developed for the treatment of AD.

AD is often labeled as extrinsic or intrinsic. When allergens penetrate the skin barrier, they may cause sensitization and increase levels of IgE. Eighty percent of patients with AD have the associated elevations in IgE, also called extrinsic AD. Twenty percent of patients do not have elevations in IgE but present with other features classic of AD. Their disease is classified as intrinsic AD. Patients with intrinsic AD have a relatively late onset, milder severity, and lack *FLG* gene defects. Patients with this subtype may have sensitization to metals such as nickel and cobalt instead of typical allergens.[20,21]

HISTORY AND EXAMINATION

When evaluating a rash for suspected AD, a thorough history of the illness is essential (**Box 1**). These questions play a vital role in making the diagnosis and evaluating for complicating factors.

Revised Hanifin criteria can assist with diagnosis (**Box 2**). Essential features include pruritus and chronic or relapsing eczematous change in a predictable distribution. This distribution can change with age. Typically, the cheeks, neck, and extensor surfaces are affected in young infants (**Fig. 1**). Flexor crease involvement is classic for any age (**Fig. 2**). The disease usually spares the inguinal crease or diaper area and axillae.

Features consistent with the diagnosis, but not exclusive, include early age of onset, xerosis, and personal or family history of atopic disease or elevated IgE.

Box 1
Taking a history

Questions for HPI:

- Age of onset
- Location and evolution of distribution
- H/o cradle cap and diaper involvement
- Exacerbating factors
- Past treatments: how much, how often, how effective?
- How often do they flare? Do they ever clear and for how long?
- Skin care regimen
- Is itch interfering with sleep, school performance, or other activities of daily living?
- Personal h/o atopy
- Family history (FH) of atopy or psoriasis
- Personal and FH of infections including streptococcal pharyngitis, staphylococcal or skin infections, herpes simplex virus, tinea, sinusitis, OM, pneumonia

Abbreviations: HPI, history of present illness; h/o, history of; OM, otitis media.

· Associated features that assist with diagnosis, but could be variable, include keratosis pilaris, pityriasis alba, hyperlinear palms and soles, ichthyosis, periorbital, perioral, and/or periauricular changes, and dermatographism.

Four features that are associated with AD and occasionally confused with AD deserve mentioning: pityriasis alba, keratosis pilaris, ichthyosis vulgaris, and dermatographism (**Fig. 3**). Pityriasis alba (PA) appears as subtle, poorly circumscribed, hypopigmented patches often preceded by fine papular change or scale. They occur most

---

Box 2
Revised Hanifin criteria, adapted for this article

- Essential features
  - Pruritus
  - Eczematous change that is chronic or relapsing in a representative pattern
    - Infants and children: face, neck, extensor surfaces
    - Infants, children, and adults: history of flexural involvement, spares inguinal crease and axillae
- Features most consistent with diagnosis but may be variable
  - Early-age at onset
  - Personal or FH of atopic disease, including elevated IgE
  - Xerosis
- Associated features aiding in diagnosis but may also be variable
  - Dermatographism
  - Keratosis pilaris, hyperlinear palms, and ichthyosis
  - Periorbital changes, including erythema, Dennie-Morgan lines, and eczematous change
  - Periauricular lesions including tendency to fissure at ear lobe creases
  - Perioral changes, including cheilitis
  - Perifollicular accentuation (more prominent in type III+ skin)
  - Lichenification and prurigo lesions often induced by scratching
- Consider comorbid and complicating conditions

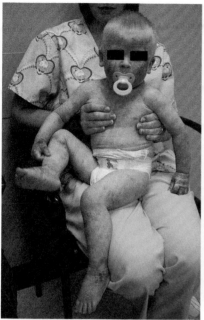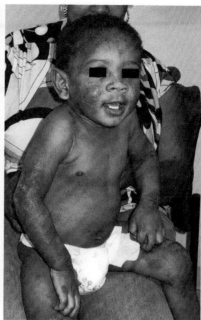

Fig. 1. Infantile distribution.

often on the face, proximal upper extremities, and occasionally trunk. Patches may be more pronounced with sun exposure as surrounding skin tans.

Keratosis pilaris is a benign disorder of family history It presents as flesh colored or erythematous, small, rough papules that are usually asymptomatic, but may cause mild pruritus. They are classically located on the upper lateral arms but may also occur on the cheeks, lower arms, gluteal prominences, and upper anterior legs.

Ichthyosis vulgaris (IV) may represent a defect in the *FLG* gene and presents as adherent, xerotic scale most easily seen on the lower legs but may affect other areas. The term ichthy means fish, referring to the fish scale appearance of the condition. It usually appears 2 to 6 months after birth, increases though puberty, and then decreases with age. The palms and soles of patients with IV are frequently hyperlinear. Approximately half of patients with IV develop AD, and the condition is associated with earlier onset and increased severity of atopic disease.[22]

Dermatographism is an immunologic response to pressure on the skin producing a wheal, then erythema or pallor, possibly followed by edema and itch. It begins within 5 minutes of stimulation and may persist for 15 to 30 minutes.[22] This tendency toward urticaria is histamine-mediated and may improve with an antihistamine.

The features associated with AD can help distinguish the disease from other conditions or comorbidities that may present in a similar fashion.

Infectious Complications

Patients with AD are prone to microbial colonization due to skin barrier dysfunction and decreased immune response to the invaders (**Box 3**, **Fig. 4**). *Staphylococcus aureus* is frequently found with skin culture but does not always indicate infection. Up to 80% to 90% of patients with AD are carriers of *S aureus*.[23] *Staphylococcus* is found on lesional and nonlesional skin in patients with AD and may trigger multiple inflammatory cascades, further damaging the epidermal barrier and potentiating atopic disease.[2,13]

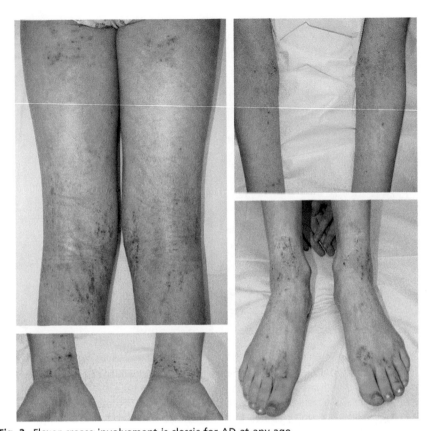

Fig. 2. Flexor crease involvement is classic for AD at any age.

If there are no signs of infection, consider treatment to reduce bacterial colonization, including dilute bleach baths. The addition of bleach to bath water can decrease microbes and may decrease inflammation. Thomas Leung and colleagues[24] demonstrated that mice with dermatitis exposed to dilute bleach baths had reductions in nuclear factor-κB, an inflammatory mediator. Therefore, dilute bleach baths may have both antimicrobial and anti-inflammatory effects.

If patients have a history of impetigo and recurrent colonization, consider mupirocin or retapamulin prophylaxis. Apply mupirocin or retapamulin to warm areas where bacteria are likely to colonize (nares and skin folds) twice a day for 5 days. Consider family members as sources of recolonization and encourage similar measures.

Bacterial infections are not as common as colonization but may complicate AD. These include impetigo, furuncles, streptococcal infections, and others. Look for classic signs of infection such as pustules or purulence, fever, malaise, and pain. A red, glossy appearance of the rash may indicate a streptococcal infection. In pediatric patients, pain can be an important symptom. If the child is no longer scratching a chronically pruritic area and instead complains of tenderness, consider infection and culture for microbes. Oral antibiotics may treat a true skin infection but do not improve or prevent an atopic flare.[25] The sensitivities provided after culture can help direct antibiotic therapy.

Viral processes can also complicate eczema. Molluscum contagiosum (MC) is a benign viral skin infection presenting as flesh colored, pink, or pearly white umbilicated

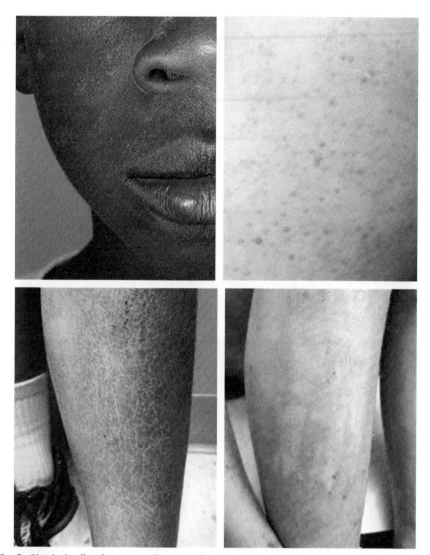

Fig. 3. Pityriasis alba, keratosis pilaris, ichthyosis vulgaris, and dermatographism.

papules. The virus can last an average of 1 to 2 years and may leave pitted scarring. In patients with AD, the virus may be more extensive and create a process known as molluscum eczema in which dermatitis develops surrounding the molluscum lesions.[22] Although there is limited evidence regarding treatment of these eruptions, consider a topical calcineurin inhibitor (TCI) rather than a topical steroid to prevent a theoretical decrease in immune response to the virus.

Eczema herpeticum (EH), is an acute-onset, potentially life-threatening viral infection caused by herpes simplex virus (HSV), occurring almost exclusively in patients with a history of chronic skin disease, especially AD.[22] Approximately 20% of patients with AD develop EH.[26] These patients have severe AD, increased atopic disease, and are more likely to have a history of S aureus or MC infections.[27] Patients present with widespread, tender, punched out erosions with a predilection for the face and areas of chronic dermatitis. Patients may also have regional lymphadenopathy. EH can be mistaken for impetigo, especially in chronic patients (EH incognito). Perform swabs for bacteria and HSV. *Staphylococcus* and *Streptococcus* may coexist with HSV. Sensitivities can be low with diagnostic procedures such as Tzanck smear, viral

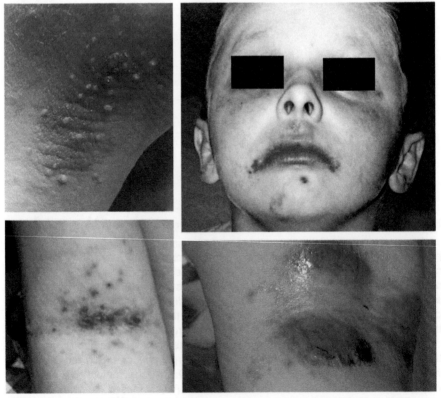

Fig. 4. Infections: molluscum contagiosum eczema, eczema herpeticum, eczema coxsackium, and streptococcal.

culture, polymerase chain reaction (PCR), or immunofluorescence, so a high index of suspicion is important. Empiric antiviral treatment may be indicated.[28]

Finally, the hand-foot-and-mouth virus can create an exacerbation known as eczema coxsackium (EC). Hand-foot-and-mouth is most often caused by coxsackie-virus A16, but a new strand that may present atypically with more generalized lesions is caused by coxsackievirus A6. EC manifests as punched out erosions or hemorrhagic vesicles in a similar manner to EH. Symptoms such as fever, rhinitis, and decreased appetite may precede the illness and, months later, onychomadesis is also associated. A diagnosis of EC is most reliably confirmed by serum PCR for coxsackievirus. Treatment is supportive, with antipyretics and bland skin care.[22]

In addition to bacterial and viral exacerbations, fungus may also invade compromised skin. Tinea may be present without its typical presentation of annular lesions with central clearing leading to tinea incognito.[22] Patients with recurrent scalp scale, persistent nummular lesions, a family history of tinea, and/or persistent AD not responsive to treatment should have a culture and/or potassium hydroxide (KOH) preparation. Oral antifungals are necessary for tinea capitis or for patients prone to contact dermatitis from topical agents.

Yeast can also complicate a presentation. Most diaper rashes in patients with skin disease are likely contact dermatitis, but infections from Candida are not uncommon.[22] Consider a culture to direct treatment. Avoid empiric topical treatment in patients prone to contact dermatitis due to the irritant or allergic potential of the ointment or cream. Consider oral agents such as fluconazole in patients with moderate to severe diaper dermatitis.

Diagnoses That May Overlap

Food allergies are seen in approximately 14% of children with mild to moderate AD and in 30% to 40% with moderate to severe disease.[29,30] The most common food allergens are cow's milk, egg, nuts, fish, and shellfish; these develop in the order exposed to the food.[31] The allergy may present as an immediate reaction, delayed eczematous reaction, or combination. Because 80% of patients with AD have elevated IgE, just the elevation does not signify a true allergy. Reproducible clinical symptoms after food exposure or ingestion are necessary to diagnose food allergy.[32] Current recommendations advise testing only for those presenting with anaphylaxis, for those who have suspicious symptoms that occur within minutes to hours of ingesting food, and for children age 5 and younger with moderate to severe disease that persists despite optimal treatment.[33] If there is consistent correlation of symptoms to food exposure, a diagnostic elimination diet of the suspected food for up to 4 to 6 weeks may be initiated.[32] If the symptoms resolve, consider avoiding the food and re-evaluating specific IgE levels periodically looking for tolerance. An IgE within normal limits is negative for food allergy. If the symptoms of AD persist after food elimination, consider re-exposure. The gold standard for assessing food allergies is a double-blind, placebo-controlled food challenge done with the help of an allergist. Fleischer and colleagues[34] completed a retrospective analysis on the outcome of oral food challenges in children with AD following elimination diets primarily based on sensitization. It demonstrated that 84% to 93% of the avoided foods were tolerated. Although food allergies may coexist and represent important triggers in a small subset of individuals with AD, the true frequency of food allergies causing an isolated flare of disease is probably low because the disease is most often multifactorial.[35] Restricting the diet may not only have implications to the child's growth but may also lead to immediate intolerance.[35] Most recently, the Learning Early about Peanut Allergy (LEAP) trial demonstrated that the early introduction of peanuts significantly decreased the frequency of the development of peanut allergy among children at high risk for this allergy.[36] The study may change the way food avoidance is recommend and is worthy of reviewing. Consensus communication notes that infants with early onset atopic disease including AD and egg allergy may benefit from early peanut exposure in the first 4 to 6 months of life with the help of an allergist.[37]

Sensitization to aeroallergens is also common in patients with AD. As previously mentioned, approximately one-third of patients with AD develop asthma and two-thirds develop allergic rhinitis.[5,6] Common aeroallergens include house dust mites, pollens, animal dander, and fungi. The role of aeroallergens in exacerbation of AD is unclear. Although patients report flares after exposure, avoidance measures and immunotherapy produce inconsistent results.[32]

The use of sedating antihistamines may be beneficial to induce sleep but have limited efficacy as an anti-itch agent because AD is not a histamine-mediated disease.[23] The exceptions are for patients who have comorbid allergic rhinitis or for those who display dermatographism or a tendency toward urticaria. These patients may benefit from a daily antihistamine.

Irritant and allergic contact dermatoses are common in patients with AD. These conditions may develop immediately or days to weeks after exposure to topical products such as soaps, lotions, cosmetics, metals, and others.

Irritant contact dermatitis is an immediate nonspecific immune response that presents as erythematous papules or plaques, edema, and/or scale in the distribution of contact. It is most common on the face, dorsal aspect of the hands, and diaper area of young children, often triggered by exposure to saliva (drooling, lip licking), urine, feces, cleansing products, and acidic or alkaline foods.[22] Avoiding the irritant can be a challenge, so application of uncomplicated zinc oxide (with inactive ingredients of petroleum jelly, mineral oil, and white wax) can act as a barrier to prevent contact with the irritant.

Patients with AD are also at risk for ACD. ACD is a delayed-type hypersensitivity response. A minimum of 10 days is required for individuals to develop specific sensitivity after the first contact, but there is a faster response after second exposure, often within 24 to 48 hours.[38] Sensitization can begin as early as 6 months with almost 25% of healthy children 6 months to 5 years having ACD.[39] Some of the more common substances that cause ACD in the general population include nickel (12.9%), cobalt (1.2%), thimerosal (9.4%), kathon/methylchloroisothiazolinone/methylisothiazolinone (2.4%), neomycin (1.2%–18.4%), and other preservatives such as formaldehyde (1.2%–13.8%).[39] In a study by Giordano-Labadie and colleagues[40] of 137 atopic children, the most frequent contact sensitizations included nickel (14.9%); fragrance (4.4%); lanolin (4.4%); balsam of Peru (2.6%); neomycin (2.6%); and emollients (2.6%) (**Box 4**). Surfactants in cleansers are also possible causes of ACD, including oleamidopropyl dimethylamine (2.3%), dimethylaminopropylamine (1.7%), and cocamidopropyl betaine (1.4%).[41] Sensitization with an allergen contained in a complex topical product can enable cosensitization to another ingredient in the same product.[22] In a patient population whose family has likely tried many over-the-counter products to control eczema, most have been exposed to multiple allergens. Because the distribution of ACD can often mimic AD, determining if ACD is playing a role in the disease can be challenging. Facial, neck, or periorbital dermatitis may suggest topical allergy to preservatives or fragrances in cosmetic products (**Fig. 5**). A periumbilical, neck, wrist, and/or earlobe dermatitis might indicate exposure to nickel or other metals.

Epicutaneous patch testing is the gold standard for the diagnosis of ACD. Patients keep patches on the back for 2 to 3 days, return to the office for initial reading, then,

Box 4
Common sources of contact allergies in atopic children

Allergen	Incidence (%)
Nickel	14.9
Fragrance	4.4
Lanolin	4.4
Balsam of Peru	2.6
Neomycin	2.6
Emollients	2.6

Data from Kwan J, Jacob S. Contact Dermatitis in the atopic child. Pediatr Ann 2012;41(10):422–3, 426–8.

due to the delayed nature of the reactions, return again several days later. The sensitivity of patch testing ranges from 60% to 80%.[32] A positive result indicates allergy, but a negative result could be a false-negative. Results can be confusing but may help give patients a better direction for treatment. Patch testing should be considered in AD patients with persistent or recalcitrant disease, and/or a history or physical examination findings consistent with ACD.[32]

Psoriasis is classically defined as erythematous plaques with silvery scale occurring on the scalp, extensor surfaces, or other sites of trauma. In infants and toddlers, the presentation is often a thinner, more pruritic plaque with less scale that occurs on the scalp, face, extensor or flexor surfaces and commonly involves the diaper area

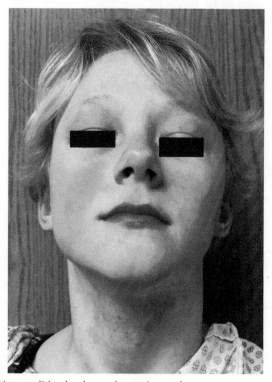

Fig. 5. ACD affecting eyelids, cheeks, and anterior neck.

(usually spared in AD). Guttate appearance is common often following an episode of *Streptococcus* infection by 1 to 3 weeks.[42] Patients may have features of both AD and psoriasis with scalp scale, flexor involvement, diaper area involvement, and focal plaques on their lower legs (**Fig. 6**). Initial treatment of the condition is similar to AD (see later discussion).

Seborrheic dermatitis is a chronic inflammatory disorder affecting areas of the head and trunk where sebaceous glands are most prominent.[43] It can present as erythematous, pruritic plaques that can mimic AD in infancy. Cradle cap and diaper area involvement may help distinguish the condition, though it is possible that the condition will overlap with AD. Washing with ketoconazole or another gentle antiyeast-medicated shampoo may decrease *Malassezia*, which is thought to contribute to the disease process. Bland skin care and anti-inflammatory agents may be necessary in more severe cases.

Infestations such as bug bites or scabies can present similarly to AD, and patients with AD may have a more brisk response to the insects or mites. Bug bites usually occur in grouped patterns on the exposed extremities more than on covered areas. Prevention with insect repellant is key. Scabies is an allergic reaction to the eggs

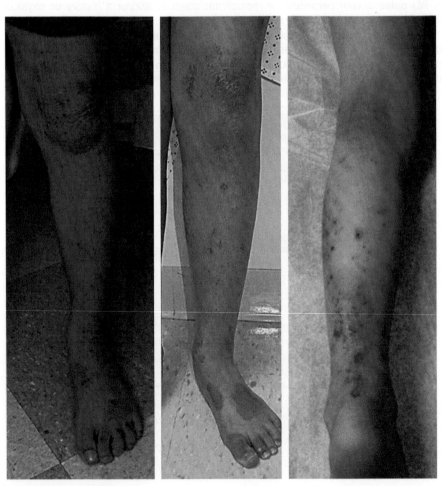

Fig. 6. Psoriasis overlap.

and feces of the female *Sarcoptes scabiei*. The reaction is characterized by small, red papules, pustules, or vesicles in a common distribution. In infants, the most commonly affected areas are palms, soles, axillae, face, and scalp. In adults, web spaces, wrists, areolar area, and genitals are most common.[22] Only those with an allergic response to the mite will have a rash, so it is important to treat all close contacts with permethrin for 10 to 12 hours repeated in 1 week. Ivermectin can be given to patients with severe skin disease at risk for contact dermatitis.

Practitioners should expand the differential if the disease is behaving atypically. There are malignancies, genetic disorders, immunodeficiencies, nutritional disorders, and other conditions that may present similarly. Consider skin biopsy, cultures, serum total IgE, patch testing, or other appropriate laboratory tests or referrals to rule out comorbidities and other skin conditions. Mimics of the disease are outside the scope of this article, but readers can consider a review of recent publications.[22,30]

TREATMENT

Because of common comorbidities and mimics of AD, diagnosis may be delayed due to the wide differential. Initial treatment, including bland skin care and anti-inflammatory measures, may make the distribution more classic and assist with diagnosis. Updated guidelines of care for the management of AD were published in the *Journal of the American Academy of Dermatology* in July 2014. Thought leaders reviewed almost 1800 abstracts and close to 250 articles. Their recommendations regarding diagnosis, assessment, treatment, and other considerations can give direction to practitioners striving to treat the disease using an evidence-based approach.[10]

Moisturization and Bland Skin Care

Because immune abnormalities and skin barrier dysfunction are present in lesional and nonlesional skin in patients with AD, several treatment recommendations are important for all patients prone to AD regardless of severity. The first is moisturization and the second is bland skin care.

Bathing is a source of confusion. It can have differing effects on the skin depending on how it is performed. Bathing with warm water for 5 to 15 minutes can hydrate the skin and remove scale, crust, irritants, and allergens.[44] Consider adding bleach to decrease microbes and possibly reduce inflammation, as previously stated. Wash with bland soaps such as Cetaphil liquid cleanser or Vanicream bar soap. Apply bland moisturizers such as petroleum jelly, mineral oil, or coconut oil directly after bathing. If the water is left to evaporate from the skin, it can have a drying effect.[45]

The ideal bland cleanser or moisturizer should be safe, effective, inexpensive, and free from preservatives, fragrances, and potential irritants or allergens. Patients and parents should read labels carefully. Soaps, lotions, and creams, even those marketed for eczema, may have added ingredients, increasing the risk of contact dermatitis. Petroleum jelly and mineral oil are moisturizers that optimize hydration without the risk of sensitization. Another alternative is coconut oil. Although there is a small risk for sensitization, a randomized, double-blind clinical trial in pediatric subjects with mild to moderate AD found superiority of virgin coconut oil over mineral oil.[46] Limit other organic oils, including olive oil. Olive oil encourages the growth of yeast and may decrease the integrity of the skin.[47,48]

Topical Steroids

Topical corticosteroids (TCSs) have been used for decades for the treatment of AD. These agents cause anti-inflammatory, antiproliferative, immunosuppressive, and vasoconstrictive effects.[49] Practitioners can consider application 1 to 2 times a day, then titrate to daily or every other day as patients regain control of a flare. After obtaining control of an outbreak, the goal is to prolong the period until the next flare. Several studies advocate the use of intermittent steroids on controlled eczema to achieve this outcome.[2]

There are a plethora of topical steroids on the market. Often, practitioners choose a lower potency steroid and increase potency as needed. The amount of medication applied can be more important than the potency. Giving patients a quantity guideline can be helpful. For example, use no more than 30 to 45 g per month. Practitioners can stratify risks by evaluating the quantities used over the course of a month. Having patients bring in the tube of the medication and calling pharmacies for refill histories will give more accurate accounts. If patients are using excessive amounts, consider a morning cortisol to screen for hypothalamic-pituitary-adrenal (HPA) axis suppression. If patients are using minimal amounts with limited efficacy, the practitioners can encourage the use of increased quantities.

Practitioners should be mindful of contact dermatitis when choosing the steroid. As previously discussed, though rare (~2%), even topical steroids can cause ACD. The most common offenders are tixocortol or hydrocortisone.[50] Because of this risk, topical steroids are divided into allergic classes A through D, including D1 and D2. Topical steroids in class D1 are the least allergenic and include agents such as betamethasone, mometasone, fluticasone, and clobetasol. Using ointments rather than creams or lotions can also decrease the risk of ACD.

Discussing side effects proactively with patients is important. Cutaneous side effects include skin atrophy, purpura, telangiectasias, striae, focal hypertrichosis, and acneiform or rosacea-like eruptions.[2] Cutaneous absorption and side-effect potential are increased by potency, thin skin, large surface areas, frequent applications, longer duration of treatment, and occlusion.[51] The risk of HPA axis suppression is low but increases with prolonged continuous use, potent strengths, and misuse, especially in individuals receiving corticosteroids concurrently in other forms (inhaled, intranasal, or oral).[52]

The patient or family may have a fear of the side effects limiting their use, which can be challenging. In a survey of 200 patients with AD, 72.5% were worried about using TCSs on their own or their child's skin, with fear of skin thinning being the most common concern, followed by long-term effects. Of those surveyed, 33% admitted that their worries stopped them from using steroids on their own or their child's skin.[53]

Another challenge to topical steroid use includes the fear of infection or impaired wound healing. A study performed using TCS application on AD lesions colonized with *S aureus* found a reduction in colonization and improvement to disease.[54] TCSs do not need to be avoided in colonized skin. Additionally, excoriated and fissured lesions should be included in treatment as the underlying inflammation and pruritus lead to these secondary changes.[2]

Topical Calcineurin Inhibitors

TCIs, tacrolimus and pimecrolimus, were introduced to the market in 2000 and 2001 and are indicated for children ages 2 to 15 years as second-line therapy for the treatment of AD in nonimmunocompromised patients who failed to respond adequately to other topical prescription treatments for AD, or when those treatments are not advisable. These topical medications are thought to inhibit the activation of T lymphocytes and subsequently decrease the release of the proinflammatory cytokines such as those implicated in AD. The most common side effects were skin burning and pruritus.[55,56]

Tacrolimus seems to be more effective than mild TCS, and pimecrolimus as effective as mild agents.[57,58] These products provide an alternative or addition to topical steroids and fulfill a niche for areas more prone to absorption and the side effects of TCS, such as the eyelids, face, flexor creases, and diaper area.

In 2006, a black box warning was added to the package inserts causing concern for many practitioners. Oral and intravenous tacrolimus administered for systemic immune suppression in transplant recipients is associated with an increased risk of immune-mediated malignancies, including lymphomas. Because of this risk, a black box warning was added to Protopic and Elidel warning that "although a causal relationship has not been established, rare cases of malignancy (eg, skin and lymphoma) have been reported in patients treated with topical calcineurin inhibitors."[55,56]

Several studies since the addition of the black box warning have shown no increases in malignancy rates relative to that of the general population.[2,58] These medications have minimal absorption, 70-fold to 100-fold less than TCS.[58,59] One such study is a longitudinal cohort study including 7457 children enrolled in the Pediatric Eczema Elective Registry (PEER) with a history of AD and use of pimecrolimus representing 26,792 person years. The results suggest that it is unlikely that topical pimecrolimus as used by the patients in the registry is associated with an increased risk of malignancy.[60]

Using TCS and TCIs in combination if appropriate may maximize effectiveness of topical therapy due to differing mechanisms of action and minimize side effects by reducing the amount of each medication needed to achieve desired results.[49,58]

As with TCS, TCIs may also reduce S aureus colonization and application to controlled areas may increase the time to the next flare.[2]

Wet Wraps

Intensive inpatient treatment with wet dressings and TCS is highly effective in controlling severe and recalcitrant AD.[61] These measures, though time consuming, can be taught at home to optimize topical treatment strategies.

SYSTEMIC THERAPIES
Phototherapy

Phototherapy is the use of ultraviolet light to treat many forms of dermatitis and inflammation. The data for use of phototherapy in children are limited but should be considered when disease is widespread or refractory to topical therapies.[62] Although there are many modalities, in-office narrowband UV-B is considered first-line phototherapy for use in children.[32] Each session lasts only a few minutes, but patients need treatments 2 to 3 times per week for several months. Most see significant improvement after 20 to 30 treatments, then maintain this response with visits 1 to 3 times per week.[62] There are obvious barriers, including scheduling, cooperation of the child, as well as possible side effects, including erythema, tenderness, stinging, HSV reactivation, skin cancer, and others. This can be an effective treatment, but an individualistic approach is necessary.

Systemic Medications

Many patients are well-controlled with bland skin care and topical medications, and the condition usually resolves before adolescence, but up to 30% of patients show a chronic, persisting course.[63] Systemic therapies are recommended when patients are not well-controlled after using safe amounts of topical medication and when complicating factors such as comorbidities are considered. There are no systemic medications approved to treat AD, but several are used off-label, including cyclosporine, methotrexate, azathioprine, mycophenolate mofetil, interferon gamma, and intravenous immunoglobulin (IVIG).

Cyclosporine is an immunosuppressant of T cells and IL-2. Taken twice a day, most patients see improvements within 2 to 6 weeks. The duration of therapy is usually limited to short courses of a few months or less due to side effects, including infection, nephrotoxicity, hypertension, tremor, hypertrichosis, headache, gingival hyperplasia, and increased risk of skin cancer and lymphoma.[23]

Methotrexate is an antifolate metabolite and blocks the synthesis of DNA, RNA, and purines. It is also thought to negatively affect T-cell function.[23] Most patients experience improvements in 2 to 3 months of therapy, but others may need dose adjustments. The most common side effects include nausea or abdominal pain, though a comprehensive metabolic panel and complete blood count should be monitored to look for elevations in liver enzymes or decreases in red and white blood cells. Pulmonary fibrosis and liver damage have also been reported. Consider supplementation with folic acid (**Fig. 7**).

Azathioprine is a purine analog that inhibits DNA production, decreasing B cells and T cells during inflammatory disease states. Side effects include nausea and vomiting at higher doses, headache, hypersensitivity reactions, elevated liver enzymes, and leukopenia. The metabolism of azathioprine depends on an individual's thiopurine methyltransferase (TPMT) activity level, a principle enzyme in the thiopurine pathway. Practitioners should get a baseline level and measure TPMT periodically during treatment.[23]

Mycophenolate mofetil blocks the de novo pathway of purine synthesis, preferentially inhibiting the proliferation of B and T cells. Adverse events (AEs) include nausea, vomiting, abdominal cramping, headache, and fatigue, and may not be dose-dependent. Rarely, cytopenia (anemia, leukopenia, and thrombocytopenia), genitourinary symptoms (urgency, frequency, dysuria), cutaneous malignancy, and lymphoma have been reported.[23]

Interferon gamma enhances natural killer cell production and increases macrophage oxidation. Because it is variably effective, it is considered alternative therapy for those with AD who did not respond to other agents.[23]

IVIG is an alternative for patients with AD and recurrent infections if immunosuppressant agents are not a good fit. Unfortunately, there is limited evidence regarding dosing and effect.[64]

If possible, systemic steroids should be avoided for the treatment of AD. Their use should be exclusively reserved for acute, severe exacerbations and as a short-term bridge therapy to other systemic, steroid-sparing therapy.[2] The effect of systemic steroid therapy is rarely sustained after discontinuation and often leads to rebound flaring despite tapering.[65]

New Therapies

As mentioned in the introduction, thought leaders have described this time period for AD as a new dawn. Phase II and III clinical trials are completed for several new agents targeting the immune abnormalities of AD. Although no therapy exists to repair the FLG gene defect, it is possible that successfully treated skin has increased expression FLG.

Dupilumab is a new therapy close to Food and Drug Administration approval. It is a fully human monoclonal antibody that is directed against the shared alpha subunit of the IL-4 receptors and blocks signaling from both IL-4 and IL-13. This is a

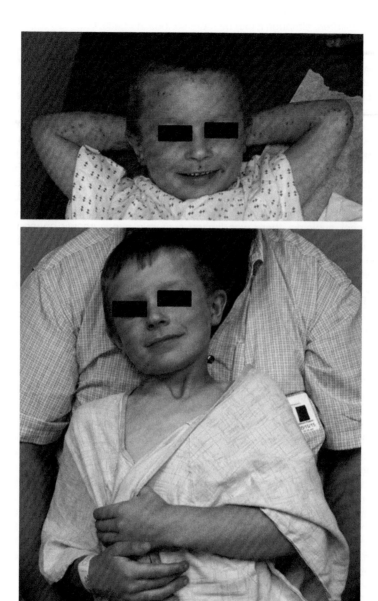

Fig. 7. Before and after 18 months methotrexate.

subcutaneous injection given once weekly. In adult subjects with moderate to severe AD not controlled with topical therapy, 85% of subjects in the dupilumab group, compared with 35% of those in the placebo group, had a 50% reduction in the Eczema Area and Severity Index (EASI) score. Forty percent of subjects in the dupilumab group, compared with 7% in the placebo group, indicated clearing or near clearing of their disease. Pruritus scores decreased by 55.7% in the dupilumab group versus 15.1% in the placebo group. The most frequent AEs in the dupilumab group were nasopharyngitis and headache. Clinical trials for pediatric subjects ages 12 to 18 years will start within the year.[66]

Another agent with promise is an anti-IL-31 receptor A antibody. IL-31 is a cytokine implicated in pruritus. A single dose of CIM331 reduced pruritus by about 50% at week 4 compared with 19.7% with placebo. CIM331 increased sleep efficiency and decreased the use of hydrocortisone butyrate.[67]

Finally, a new topical medication is on the horizon. Crisaborole 2% ointment is a boron-based topical phosphodiesterase E−4 (PDE4) inhibitor. PDE4 is an enzyme involved in the proinflammatory cascade. The agent also reduces the production of tumor necrosis factor (TNF)-alpha. In adults with mild to moderate AD, 68% of subjects experienced a greater decrease in the Atopic Dermatitis Severity Index score in lesions treated with crisaborole 2% ointment than in lesions treated with vehicle. No serious or severe AEs were reported, and no subject discontinued due to an AE.[68] In adolescent subjects, there was limited systemic exposure and mean treatable body surface area declined from 17.6% to 8.2%.[69] This may serve as an alternative or addition to other topical medications.

One agent that is already approved for rheumatoid arthritis may also benefit patients with AD. Tofacitinib is a Janus kinase inhibitor and in a small trial of 6 subjects with severe AD, the AD index score decreased by 66%. There were no AEs.[70]

There are other molecules in development that may target additional cytokines implicated in AD. The landscape for treatment is changing dramatically and possibilities are exciting.

SUMMARY

In the last decade, huge strides were made in understanding the pathogenesis of AD. There are new molecules that could revolutionize the way disease is treated and may have impacts on other atopic and inflammatory conditions. Although these therapies may not have pediatric approval for some years, the current models explaining skin barrier defects and immune abnormalities can be used to optimize current treatment. Early diagnosis and treatment may help limit the morbidity of the disease and could prevent or limit the severity of other atopic diseases. The cornerstone of treatment is moisturization of lesional and nonlesional skin and bland skin care. Addressing inflammation with the appropriate topical steroid, then adding a TCI when needed can optimize skin barrier function and target immune abnormalities. Consider microbes, comorbidities, and other mimics when the disease is behaving atypically. AD can ruin a patient's life if left uncontrolled, but practitioners can maximize current treatment options to limit the morbidity.

REFERENCES

1. Shaw TE, Currie GP, Koudelka CW, et al. Eczema prevalence in the United States: data from the 2003 National Survey of Children's Health. J Invest Dermatol 2011; 131:67–73.
2. Eichenfield LF, Tom WL, Berger TG, et al. Guidelines of care for the management of atopic dermatitis: section 2. Management and treatment of atopic dermatitis with topical therapies. J Am Acad Dermatol 2014;71(1):116–32.
3. CenterWatch. FDA approved drugs for dermatology. Boston, MA: CenterWatch; 1995–2016. Available at: https://www.centerwatch.com/drug-information/fda-approved-drugs/therapeutic-area/3/dermatology. Accessed December 30, 2015.
4. Thomsen SF. Epidemiology and natural history of atopic disease. Eur Clin Respir J 2015;2. http://dx.doi.org/10.3402/ecrj.v2.24642.

5. van der Hulst AE, Klip H, Brand PL. Risk of developing asthma in young children with atopic eczema: a systemic review. J Allergy Clin Immunol 2007;120:565–9.

6. Spergel JM. Epidemiology of atopic dermatitis and atopic march in children. Immunol Allergy Clin N Am 2010;30:269–80.

7. Bieber T. Atopic dermatitis. Ann Dermatol 2010;22(2):125–37.

8. Gittler JK, Krueger JG, Guttman-Yassky E. Atopic dermatitis results in intrinsic barrier and immune abnormalities: implications for contact dermatitis. J Allergy Clin Immunol 2013;131(2):300–13.

9. Garg N, Silverberg J. Epidemiology of childhood atopic dermatitis. Clin Dermatol 2015;22:281–8.

10. Eichenfield LF, Tom WL, Chamlin SL, et al. Guidelines of care for the management of atopic dermatitis: Part 1: diagnosis and assessment of atopic dermatitis. J Am Acad Dermatol 2014;70(2):338–51.

11. DaVeiga SP. Epidemiology of atopic dermatitis: a review. Allergy Asthma Proc 2012;33(3):227–34.

12. Flohr C, Yeo L. Atopic dermatitis and the hygiene hypothesis revisited. Curr Probl Dermatol 2011;41:1–34.

13. Leung D, Guttman-Yassky E. Deciphering the complexities of atopic dermatitis: shifting paradigms in treatment approaches. J Allergy Clin Immunol 2014; 134(4):769–79.

14. McLean WHI. The allergy gene. Scientist 2010. Available at: http://www.the-scientist.com/?articles.view/articleNo/29383/title/The-Allergy-Gene. Accessed February 21, 2016.

15. Sandilands A, Sutherland C, Irvine A, et al. Filaggrin in the frontline: role in skin barrier function and disease. J Cell Sci 2009;122(9):1285–94.

16. U.S. National Library of Medicine. FLG. Genetics Home Reference. 2016. Available at: http://ghr.nlm.nih.gov/gene/FLG. Accessed February 29, 2016.

17. McLean I, Irvine A. Heritable filaggrin disorders: the paradigm of atopic dermatitis. J Invest Dermatol 2012;132(Suppl 3):E20–1.

18. Irvine A, McLean I, Leung D. Filaggrin mutations associated with skin and allergic diseases. N Engl J Med 2011;365:1315–27.

19. Leung D, Guttman-Yassky E. Deciphering the complexities of atopic dermatitis: Shifting paradigms in treatment approaches. J Allergy Clin Immunol 2014; 13(4):769–79.

20. Tokura Y. Extrinsic and intrinsic types of atopic dermatitis. J Dermatol Sci 2010; 58(1):1–7.

21. Yamaguchi H, Kabashima-Kubo R, Bito T, et al. High frequencies of positive nickel/cobalt patch tests and high sweat nickel concentration in patients with intrinsic atopic dermatitis. J Dermatol Sci 2013;72:240–5.

22. Siegfried EC, Hebert AA. Diagnosis of atopic dermatitis: Mimics, overlaps, and complications. J Clin Med 2015;4:884–917.

23. Sidbury R, Davis D, Cohen D, et al. Guidelines of care for the management of atopic dermatitis, Part 3:Management and treatment with phototherapy and systemic agents. J Am Acad Dermatol 2014;71(2):327–49.

24. Leung T, Zhang L, Wang J, et al. Topical hypochlorite ameliorates NF-κB–mediated skin diseases in mice. J Clin Invest 2013;123(12):5361–70.

25. Berke R, Singh A, Guralnick M. Atopic dermatitis: an overview. Am Fam Physician 2012;86(1):35–42.

26. Peng WM, Jenneck C, Bussmann C, et al. Risk factors of atopic dermatitis patients for eczema herpeticum. J Invest Dermatol 2007;127:1261–3.

27. Beck LA, Boguniewicz M, Hata T, et al. Phenotype of atopic dermatitis subjects with a history of eczema herpeticum. J Allergy Clin Immunol 2009;124:260–9.
28. Frisch S, Siegfried EC. The clinical spectrum and therapeutic challenge of eczema herpeticum. Pediatr Dermatol 2011;28:46–52.
29. Wassmann A, Werfel T. Atopic eczema and food allergy. Chem Immunol Allergy 2015;101:181–90.
30. Awasthi S, Rothe M, Eichenfield L. Atopic dermatitis: kids are not just little people. Clin Dermatol 2015;33(6):594–604.
31. Boyce JA, Assa'ad A, Burks AW, et al. Guidelines for the diagnosis and management of food allergy in the United States: report of the NIAID-sponsored expert panel. J Allergy Clin Immunol 2010;126:S1–58.
32. Sidbury R, Tom W, Bergmen J, et al. Guidelines of care for the management of atopic dermatitis part 4: prevention of disease flares and use of adjunctive therapies and approaches. J Am Acad Dermatol 2014;71(6):1218–33.
33. Burks AW, Jones SM, Boyce JA, et al. NIAID-sponsored 2010 guidelines for managing food allergy: Applications in the pediatric population. Pediatrics 2011;128: 955–65.
34. Fleischer DM, Bock SA, Spears GC, et al. Oral food challenges in children with a diagnosis of food allergy. J Pediatr 2011;158:578–83.
35. Chang A, Robinson R, Cai M, et al. Natural history of food-triggered atopic dermatitis and development of immediate reactions in children. J Allergy Clin Immunol Pract 2015. http://dx.doi.org/10.1016/j.jaip.2015.08.006.
36. DuToit G, Roberts G, Sayre PH, et al. Randomized trial of peanut consumption in infants at risk for peanut allergy. N Engl J Med 2015;372:803–13.
37. Fleischer D, Sicherer S, Greenhawt M, et al. Consensus communication on early peanut introduction and the prevention of peanut allergy in high-risk infants. Pediatr Dermatol 2016;33(1):103–6.
38. Hogan D. Irritant contact dermatitis treatment and management. Medscape. Available at: http://emedicine.medscape.com/article/1049353-treatment#aw2aab6b6b4. Accessed November 8, 2012.
39. Bruckner A, Weston W, Morelli G. Does sensitization to contact allergens begin in infancy? Pediatrics 2000;105(1):e3.
40. Kwan J, Jacob S. Contact dermatitis in the atopic child. Pediatr Ann 2012;41(10): 422–3, 426–8.
41. Fowler J, Shaughnessy C, Belsito D, et al. Cutaneous delayed-type hypersensitivity to surfactants. Dermatitis 2014;26(6):268–70.
42. Tollefson M, Crowson C, McEvoy M, et al. Incidence of psoriasis in children: a population-based study. J Am Acad Dermatol 2010;62(6):979–87.
43. Johnson B, Nunley J. Treatment of seborrheic dermatitis. Am Fam Physician 2000;61(9):2703–10.
44. Gutman AB, Kligman AM, Sciacca J, et al. Soak and smear: a standard technique revisited. Arch Dermatol 2005;141:1556–9.
45. Chiang C, Eichenfield LF. Quantitative assessment of combination bathing and moisturizing regimens on skin hydration in atopic dermatitis. Pediatr Dermatol 2009;26:273–8.
46. Evangelista MT, Abad-Casintahan F, Lopez-Villafuerte L. The effect of topical virgin coconut oil on SCORAD index, transepidermal water loss, and skin capacitance in mild to moderate pediatric atopic dermatitis: a randomized, double-blind, clinical trial. Int J Dermatol 2014;53(1):100–8.
47. Siegfried E, Glenn E. Use of olive oil for the treatment of seborrheic dermatitis in children. Arch Pediatr Adolesc Med 2012;166(10):967.

48. Danby S, AlEnezi T, Sultan A, et al. Effect of olive and sunflower oil on the adult skin barrier: implications for neonatal skin care. Pediatr Dermatol 2013;30(1). 42–50.

49. Norris DA. Mechanisms of action of topical therapies and rationale for combination therapy. J Am Acad Dermatol 2005;53:S17–25.

50. Vind-Kezunovic D, Johansen JD, Carlsen BC. Prevalence of and factors influencing sensitization to corticosteroids in a Danish patch test population. Contact Dermatitis 2011;64(6):325–9.

51. Morley KW, Dinulos JG. Update on topical glucocorticoid use in children. Curr Opin Pediatr 2012;24(1):121–8.

52. Ellison JA, Patel L, Ray DW, et al. Hypothalamic-pituitary-adrenal function and glucocorticoid sensitivity in atopic dermatitis. Pediatrics 2000;105:794–9.

53. Charman CR, Morris AD, Williams HC. Topical corticosteroid phobia in patients with atopic eczema. Br J Dermatol 2000;142:931–6.

54. Gong JQ, Lin L, Lin T, et al. Skin colonization by *Staphylococcus aureus* in patients with eczema and atopic dermatitis and relevant coined topical therapy: a double-blind multicenter randomized controlled trial. Br J Dermatol 2006;155: 680–7.

55. Protopic® (Tacrolimus) ointment 0.03 % and ointment 0.1 % (US prescribing information). Deerfield (IL): Astellas Pharma US, Inc.; 2011.

56. Elidel® (Pimecrolimus) cream 1 % (US prescribing information). East Hanover (NJ): Novartis Pharmaceuticals Corporation; 2010.

57. Ashcroft DM, Dimmock P, Garside R, et al. Efficacy and tolerability of topical pimecrolimus and tacrolimus in the treatment of atopic dermatitis: meta-analysis of randomised controlled trials. BMJ 2005;330(7490):516.

58. Carr WW. Topical calcineurin inhibitors for atopic dermatitis: review and treatment recommendations. Paediatr Drugs 2013;15(4):303–10.

59. Stuetz A, Baumann K, Grassgerger M, et al. Discovery of topical calcineurin inhibitors and pharmacological profile of pimecrolimus. Int Arch Allergy Immunol 2006;141(3):199–212.

60. Margolis DJ, Abuabara K, Hoffstad OJ, et al. Association Between Malignancy and Topical Use of Pimecrolimus. JAMA Dermatol 2015;151(6):594–9.

61. Dabade T, Davis D, Wetter D, et al. Wet dressing therapy in conjunction with topical corticosteroids is effective for rapid control of severe pediatric atopic dermatitis: experience with 218 patients over 30 years at Mayo Clinic. J Am Acad Dermatol 2012;67(1):100–6.

62. Song E, Reja D, Silverberg N, et al. Phototherapy: Kids are not just little people. Clin Dermatol 2015;33(6):672–80.

63. Lauffer F, Ring J. Target-oriented therapy: Emerging drugs for atopic dermatitis. Expert Opin Emerg Drugs 2016;21(1):81–9.

64. Turner P, Kakakios A, Wong L, et al. Intravenous immunoglobulin to treat severe atopic dermatitis in children: a case series. Pediatr Dermatol 2012;29(2):177–81.

65. Schmitt J, Schakel K, Folster-Holst R, et al. Prednisolone vs. ciclosporin for severe adult eczema. An investigator-initiated double-blind placebo-controlled multicentre trial. Br J Dermatol 2010;162:661–8.

66. Beck L, Thaci D, Hamilton J, et al. Dupilumab treatments in adults with moderate-to-severe atopic dermatitis. N Engl J Med 2014;371(2):130–9.

67. Nemoto O, Furue M, Nakagawa H, et al. The first trial of CIM331, a humanized anti-human IL-31 receptor A antibody, for healthy volunteers and patients with atopic dermatitis to evaluate safety, tolerability and pharmacokinetics of a single

dose in a randomised, double-blind, placebo-controlled study. Br J Dermatol 2016;174(2):296–304.

68. Murrell D, Gebauer K, Spelman L, et al. Crisaborole topical ointment, 2% in adults with atopic dermatitis: a phase 2a, vehicle-controlled, proof-of-concept study. J Drugs Dermatol 2015;14(10):1108–12.

69. Tom W, VanSyoc M, Chanda S, et al. Pharmacokinetic profile, safety, and tolerability of crisaborole topical ointment, 2% in adolescents with atopic dermatitis: An open-label phase 2a study. Pediatr Dermatol 2016. http://dx.doi.org/10.1111/pde.12780.

70. Levy L, Urban J, King B. Treatment of recalcitrant atopic dermatitis with the oral Janus kinase inhibitor tofacitinib citrate. J Am Acad Dermatol 2015;73(3):395–9.

Attention-Deficit/ Hyperactivity Disorder

An Update for the Pediatric Primary Care Provider

Courtney F. Andrus, MMS, PA-C, RD, LD

KEYWORDS

- Attention-deficit/hyperactivity disorder • Pediatric mental health
- Stimulant medication • Medical management of ADHD

KEY POINTS

- Attention-deficit/hyperactivity disorder (ADHD) is the most common pediatric mental health disorder, and the prevalence continues to increase.
- Most patients have comorbid mental health conditions that either manifest as ADHD or complicate the diagnosis of ADHD.
- ADHD is a chronic medical condition, often persisting into adulthood. Primary care pediatricians must recognize ADHD and initiate therapy in a timely manner to reduce the risk of misdiagnosed or poorly managed adulthood ADHD, which can lead to substance abuse, failure in the workplace, poor socialization, and peer problems.
- Stimulant medications remain first-line therapy for the management of ADHD. However, clinicians can also consider nonstimulant medications, behavior therapy, and medical nutrition therapy for the primary or supplemental treatment of ADHD.

INTRODUCTION

Attention-deficit/hyperactivity disorder (ADHD) is the most common neurobehavioral disorder in childhood and adolescence and has an estimated worldwide prevalence of approximately 3.4% to 7.2%.[1,2] ADHD is a consistent pattern of behaviors causing the inability to maintain sustained attention and focus and increased impulsivity that affects an individual in multiple settings.[3] There has been a 42% increase in the diagnosis of childhood ADHD from the years 2004 to 2012.[4] This places a financial and social burden on society as the cost of health care continues to rise and mental health care becomes more limited.[5] The Diagnostic and Statistical Manual of Mental Disorders (DSM), sets guidelines for the diagnosis of mental health disorders. The 5th edition, released in May 2013, was its first major revision since 1994.[6] Primary care

The author has nothing to disclose.
University Pediatric Associates, LLC, Washington University School of Medicine, 13001 North Outer Forty Road, Suite 310, St. Louis, MO 63017, USA
E-mail address: andrusc@wudosis.wustl.edu

Physician Assist Clin 1 (2016) 683–699
http://dx.doi.org/10.1016/j.cpha.2016.06.001
2405-7991/16/$ – see front matter © 2016 Elsevier Inc. All rights reserved.
physicianassistant.theclinics.com

providers (PCPs) are on the front-line for the screening and diagnosis of ADHD, diagnosing nearly 53.1% of cases.[7] This article provides an update for pediatric PCPs (physicians, physician assistants, and nurse practitioners) on the screening, diagnosis, and management of ADHD in children and adolescents.

ATTENTION-DEFICIT/HYPERACTIVITY DISORDER BACKGROUND
Definition

ADHD is a neurobehavioral condition primarily affecting children but often persisting into adolescence and adulthood. The symptoms must present in multiple settings (ie, home, school, work); be inappropriate for developmental level; and interfere with the individual's level of functioning, social development, learning processes, and quality of life.[4,8] There are three presentations of ADHD: (1) inattentive, (2) hyperactive, and (3) combined.[8,9] The DSM-V lists the criteria used to determine the ADHD presentation (**Box 1**).[3,6,8–10]

Diagnostic and Statistical Manual of Mental Disorders-IV Versus Diagnostic and Statistical Manual of Mental Disorders-V

The DSM revisions more broadly classify ADHD as a chronic disorder so clinicians can better recognize and manage adulthood ADHD (**Box 2**).[3] The DSM-V liberalizes the diagnostic criteria of ADHD by raising the age of symptom onset, reducing the severity of clinical impairment, and reducing the number of criteria met by adolescents and adults. Because of these revisions, the prevalence of ADHD will continue to increase as more children, adolescents, and adults meet the diagnostic criteria.[6]

Prevalence

The worldwide prevalence of ADHD continues to increase.[11] The US prevalence of children diagnosed with ADHD was 7.8%, 9.5%, and 11% in 2003, 2007, and 2011 respectively, representing nearly 6.4 million children.[4] Compared with 2003, in 2011 there were nearly 2 million more children diagnosed with ADHD and 1 million more children prescribed medication for ADHD.[4] The number of visits to ambulatory care centers for evaluation and management of ADHD is increasing, according to analyses of insurance claims filed between 2001 and 2010, although this may not represent the uninsured.[4]

The prevalence of ADHD is higher in boys with an estimated male/female ratio between 4:1 and 9:1.[12,13] The median age for diagnosis is 7 years old, with one-third of total children being diagnosed before age 6 years.[7] The inattentive type is the most common presentation.[9]

The prevalence is increasing for several reasons. Increased awareness and social acceptance of the disorder give parents and teachers confidence to request behavioral evaluations for their children or students.[4,12] Improved screening tools and PCP knowledge increase diagnosis rates.[4,12] More sophisticated health care has improved the survival of infants who are at increased risk for neurobehavioral disorders.[12]

This increased prevalence greatens the societal need for mental health, education, and social services and demands PCPs assume the responsibility of assessment and management of this chronic disorder.[12]

Pathophysiology

In theory, an imbalance of neurotransmitters, dopamine and noradrenaline, may cause ADHD. These neurotransmitters strengthen the attention of the prefrontal cortex, the part of the brain assumed responsible for executing high levels of functioning, such as organizing, prioritizing tasks, and maintaining mood.[14,15] Neurotransmitter imbalance

---

Box 1

DSM-V Diagnostic Criteria for Attention-Deficit/Hyperactivity Disorder

A. A persistent pattern of inattention and/or hyperactivity-impulsivity that interferes with functioning or development, as characterized by (1) and/or (2):

1. Inattention: Six (or more) of the following symptoms have persisted for at least 6 months to a degree that is inconsistent with developmental level and that negatively impacts directly on social and academic/occupational activities. Note: The symptoms are not solely a manifestation of oppositional behavior, defiance, hostility, or failure to understand tasks or instructions. For older adolescents and adults (age 17 and older), at least five symptoms are required.

   a. Often fails to give close attention to details or makes careless mistakes in schoolwork, at work, or during other activities (eg, overlooks or misses details, work is inaccurate).

   b. Often has difficulty sustaining attention in tasks or play activities (eg, has difficulty remaining focused during lectures, conversations, or lengthy reading).

   c. Often does not seem to listen when spoken to directly (eg, mind seems elsewhere, even in the absence of any obvious distraction).

   d. Often does not follow through on instructions and fails to finish schoolwork, chores, or duties in the workplace (eg, starts tasks but quickly loses focus and is easily sidetracked).

   e. Often has difficulty organizing tasks and activities (eg, difficulty managing sequential tasks; difficulty keeping materials and belongings in order; messy, disorganized work; has poor time management; fails to meet deadlines).

   f. Often avoids, dislikes, or is reluctant to engage in tasks that require sustained mental effort (eg, schoolwork or homework; for older adolescents and adults, preparing reports, completing forms, reviewing lengthy papers).

   g. Often loses things necessary for tasks or activities (eg, school materials, pencils, books, tools, wallets, keys, paperwork, eyeglasses, mobile telephones).

   h. Is often easily distracted by extraneous stimuli (for older adolescents and adults, may include unrelated thoughts).

   i. Is often forgetful in daily activities (eg, doing chores, running errands; for older adolescents and adults, returning calls, paying bills, keeping appointments).

2. Hyperactivity and impulsivity: Six (or more) of the following symptoms have persisted for at least 6 months to a degree that is inconsistent with developmental level and that negatively impacts directly on social and academic/occupational activities. Note: The symptoms are not solely a manifestation of oppositional behavior, defiance, hostility, or a failure to understand tasks or instructions. For older adolescents and adults (age 17 and older), at least five symptoms are required.

   a. Often fidgets with or taps hands or feet or squirms in seat.

   b. Often leaves seat in situations where remaining seated is expected (eg, leaves his or her place in the classroom, in the office or other workplace, or in other situations that require remaining in place.)

   c. Often runs about or climbs in situations where it is inappropriate (in adolescents or adults, may be limited to feeling restless).

   d. Often unable to play or engage in leisure activities quietly.

   e. Is often "on the go," acting as if "driven by a motor" (eg, is unable to be or uncomfortable being still for extended time, as in restaurants, meetings; may be experienced by others as being restless or difficult to keep up with).

   f. Often talks excessively.

   g. Often blurts out an answer before a question has been completed (eg, completes people's sentences; cannot wait for turn in conversation).

   h. Often has difficulty waiting his or her turn (eg, while waiting in line).

   i. Often interrupts or intrudes on others (eg, butts into conversations, games, or activities; may start using other people's things without asking or receiving permission; for adolescents and adults, may intrude into or take over what others are doing).

B. Several inattention or hyperactive-impulsive symptoms were present before age 12 years.

C. Several inattentive or hyperactive-impulsive symptoms are present in two or more settings (eg, at home, school, or work; with friends or relatives; in other activities).

D. There is clear evidence that the symptoms interfere with, or reduce the quality of, social, academic, or occupational functioning.

E. The symptoms do not occur exclusively during the course of schizophrenia or another psychotic disorder and are not better explained by another mental disorder (eg, mood disorder, anxiety disorder, dissociative disorder, personality disorder, substance intoxication or withdrawal).

Specify whether:
   314.01 (F90.2) Combined presentation: If both Criterion A1 (inattention) and Criterion A2 (hyperactivity-impulsivity) are met for the past 6 months.
   314.00 (F90.0) Predominantly inattentive presentation: If Criterion A1 (inattention) is met but Criterion A2 (hyperactivity-impulsivity) is not met for the past 6 months.
   314.01 (F90.1) Predominantly hyperactive/impulsive presentation: If Criterion A2 (hyperactivity-impulsivity) is met and Criterion A1 (inattention) is not met for the past 6 months.

Specify if:
   In partial remission: When full criteria were previously met, fewer than the full criteria have been met for the past 6 months, and the symptoms still result in impairment in social, academic, or occupational functioning.

Specify current severity:
   Mild: Few, if any, symptoms in excess of those required to make the diagnosis are present, and symptoms result in no more than minor impairments in social or occupational functioning.
   Moderate: Symptoms or functional impairment between "mild" and "severe" are present.
   Severe: Many symptoms in excess of those required to make the diagnosis, or several symptoms that are particularly severe, are present, or the symptoms result in marked impairment in social or occupational functioning.

Other Specified Attention-Deficit/Hyperactivity Disorder: 314.01 (F90.8)
   This category applies to presentations in which symptoms characteristic of attention-deficit/ hyperactivity disorder that cause clinically significant distress or impairment in social, occupational, or other important areas of functioning predominate but do not meet the full criteria for attention-deficit/hyperactivity disorder or any of the disorders in the neurodevelopmental disorders diagnostic class. The other specified attention-deficit/ hyperactivity disorder category is used in situations in which the clinician chooses to communicate the specific reason that the presentation does not meet the criteria for attention-deficit/hyperactivity disorder or any specific neurodevelopmental disorder. This is done by recording "other specified attention-deficit/hyperactivity disorder" followed by the specific reason (eg, "with insufficient inattention symptoms").

Unspecified Attention-Deficit/Hyperactivity Disorder: 314.01 (F90.9)
   This category applies to presentations in which symptoms characteristic of attention-deficit/ hyperactivity disorder that cause clinically significant distress or impairment in social, occupational, or other important areas of functioning predominate but do not meet the full criteria for attention-deficit/hyperactivity disorder or any of the disorders in the neurodevelopmental disorders diagnostic class. The unspecified attention-deficit/ hyperactivity disorder category is used in situations in which the clinician chooses *not* to specify the reason that the criteria are not met for attention-deficit/hyperactivity disorder or for a specific neurodevelopmental disorder, and includes presentations in which there is insufficient information to make a more specific diagnosis.

From the Diagnostic and statistical manual of mental disorders, 5th edition. Arlington, VA; American Psychiatric Association; 2013; with permission.

| Box 2
Comparison between DSM-IV and DSM V		
	DSM-IV	**DSM-V**
Age of symptom onset	Before age 7 y	Before age 12 y
Impairment of symptoms to an individual's quality of life	Symptoms must cause clinically *significant* impairment to level of functioning in two or more settings	Symptoms must be present but *do not need to significantly* impair functioning in two or more settings
Descriptive examples of symptoms listed	No	Yes
Symptom criteria in adolescents and adults (17 y and older)	Six criteria symptoms must be met for a diagnosis	Five criteria symptoms must be met for a diagnosis

Data from American Psychiatric Association. DSM-5 attention deficit/hyperactivity disorder fact sheet. Arlington, VA: American Psychiatric Publishing; 2013. Available at: http://www.dsm5.org/documents/adhd%20fact%20sheet.pdf. Accessed December 5, 2015; and Rabiner D. New diagnostic criteria for ADHD: subtle but important changes. In: Attention research update. 2013. Available at: http://www.helpforadd.com/2013/june.htm. Accessed December 17, 2015.

is speculated to cause physical changes to brain matter as evidenced by functional MRI and diffusion tensor imaging.[16]

Etiology

The exact cause of ADHD in childhood is incompletely understood and likely multifactorial.[8] It is one of the most heritable psychiatric disorders.[17] First-degree relatives of individuals with ADHD have a five- to six-fold greater risk of being affected with ADHD when compared with the general population.[16] Monozygotic twins show a nearly 79% concordance rate for ADHD compared with only 32% in same-gender dizygotic twins.[16] Rare gene variants found in some individuals with ADHD are also found in individuals with autism, schizophrenia, and Tourette syndrome.[18] More studies are needed to clarify if these gene variants directly cause ADHD or if they just predispose the carrier to developing a behavioral disorder in a certain environment.

Several environmental factors increase overall risk of developing ADHD: maternal alcohol and drug use, low socioeconomic status, younger or older parental age at time of conception, the use of assisted reproductive technologies, and multiple births.[12,16] These are also risks for poor fetal growth and prematurity.[2] Clinicians speculate whether these environmental risk factors directly cause neurobehavioral disorders and ADHD, or if they increase the infant's risk of prematurity, which indirectly increases the likelihood of a child developing ADHD.

Nutritional deficiencies, particularly of iron, zinc, magnesium, and long-chain polyunsaturated fatty acids (PUFAs), are associated with the development and worsening of childhood ADHD symptoms.[19]

EVALUATION AND DIAGNOSIS

ADHD evaluations in the primary care office include interviewing the patient and parents, reviewing screening forms, and conducting a physical examination. A complete prenatal history and a complete family history of neurobehavioral and cardiac disorders should be obtained.

Behavior reports from parents and teachers are required.[8] Standardized screening forms assessing inattention, hyperactivity, and comorbid disorders are effective.[20]

Although several screening tools are available, not one is the gold standard.[8] The most commonly used in the primary care setting, Conners 3rd Edition (Conners) and Vanderbilt Attention-Deficit Hyperactivity Disorder Diagnostic Rating Scale (Vanderbilt), are discussed here.

Diagnostic Tools

The Conners scales are available for parents and teachers and are validated for the screening of ADHD, oppositional defiant disorder, and conduct disorder in children ages 6 to 18 years.[21] They have been used for several decades and have a sensitivity of 78% and specificity of 91% for determining children with ADHD.[8]

The Vanderbilt assessment scales for parents and teachers screen for ADHD, oppositional defiant disorder, conduct disorder, anxiety, depression, and associated performance impairment in children ages 6 to 12 years old.[22,23] The Vanderbilt teacher screen has a sensitivity of 63% and a specificity of 78% for determining children with ADHD.[24] The Vanderbilt is endorsed by the American Academy of Pediatrics because of its ability to comprehensively screen for comorbid conditions and its ease of use by respondents and clinicians.[22,23]

Assessment scales are reliable screening tools for ADHD, but are not sufficient for a diagnosis. Clinical interview and meeting the DSM-V criteria are necessary to confirm the diagnosis (see **Box 1**).

Differential Diagnosis

ADHD can often be misdiagnosed or undiagnosed because of coexisting conditions.[1,16,20,25] Before making the diagnosis of ADHD, several conditions should be ruled out. A vision and hearing screen must be completed. A child with a visual or auditory deficit is less likely to remain focused, which may be falsely diagnosed as an inattention disorder. The provider must obtain a detailed sleep history because children with sleep deprivation have more daytime hyperactivity, impulsivity, and inattention.[13] Learning disorders may be mistaken as inattention. Children and adolescents with depression, anxiety, or substance abuse have poor focus and can be inappropriately diagnosed with inattention or hyperactivity disorders.[26]

Comorbid Conditions

Approximately 75% of children with ADHD have at least one comorbid psychiatric disorder, and nearly 20% of children have three or more.[13,27] These include depression, anxiety, conduct disorder, antisocial personality disorders, and sleep disorders.[1,16,20,25] Oppositional defiant disorder is seen in almost 50% of ADHD cases, making it the most common comorbid condition.[20] Children and adolescents with ADHD are nearly 2.5 times more likely to have a substance abuse disorder and are more likely to engage in high-risk sexual behaviors when compared with peers without ADHD.[26,28] Nearly 12% of children with ADHD suffer from depression.[29] PCPs must consider comorbid conditions, because it may alter the child's response to treatment of ADHD.[1] Children with comorbidities suffer more impairment than those without comorbidities.[20,27]

MANAGEMENT

The neurotransmitter imbalance can be successfully managed with medications, behavioral interventions, and nutritional therapy. The goal is to manage the symptoms of ADHD while limiting side effects.[1] Management depends on the child's age and severity of symptoms (**Box 3**).[1]

Box 3	
Recommended management of ADHD by age	
Age	**Recommended Management**
Preschool (4–5 y)	Primary: behavior therapy
	Secondary: methylphenidate (off-label)
Elementary school age (6–11 y)	Primary: FDA-approved medication
	Secondary: behavior therapy (preferably both)
Adolescents (11–18 y)	Primary: FDA-approved medication
	Secondary: behavior therapy (preferably both)

Abbreviation: FDA, Food and Drug Administration.

Data from Subcommittee on attention-deficit/hyperactivity disorder, steering committee on quality improvement and management. ADHD: clinical practice guideline for the diagnosis, evaluation, and treatment of attention-deficit/hyperactivity disorder in children and adolescents. Pediatrics 2011;128:1007–22.

Medication Therapy

Medication therapy is the mainstay of ADHD treatment in children 6 years and older.[4] The number of prescriptions has consistently increased since first becoming approved for medical use by the Food and Drug Administration (FDA) in the 1960s.[30] However, approximately 30% of children diagnosed with ADHD remain unmedicated.[31] Medications are classified as either stimulants or nonstimulants. **Table 1** lists approved medications for ADHD management.

Stimulants

Stimulant medications are the most well-studied psychopharmacologics in the pediatric population. Amphetamines and methylphenidates were determined effective at improving ADHD symptoms in the 1930s and 1950s, respectively.[14] FDA-approved stimulant medications are the first-line treatment of ADHD in children 6 years and older, with long-acting methylphenidate being the recommended starting drug.[4,32] Stimulant medications demonstrate an overall positive response rate of approximately 65% to 75%.[14] The use of methylphenidate in children younger than 6 years is more appropriately managed by a child psychiatrist or neurologist because of the difficulty in making the diagnosis in very young children.

Pharmacology Stimulant medications work by stimulating catecholamine transmission in the cerebral cortex thus increasing the availability of certain neurotransmitters in the synaptic cleft, primarily dopamine and noradrenaline.[14,16,26] Amphetamines primarily promote the release of these neurotransmitters into the synaptic cleft and secondarily block their reuptake.[14] Methylphenidates primarily block their reuptake.[14] By doing so, stimulant medications improve impulsivity, inattention, and executive functioning, which subsequently enhances academic performance, peer relationships, aggression, and mood disorders.[14]

Amphetamines and methylphenidates are available in long-acting and short-acting formulations. Long-acting medications release the active ingredient in a time-released mechanism over an average of 8 to 12 hours. Short-acting medications release the active ingredient immediately and provide symptom control for an average of 4 to 6 hours.

The clinician determines which medication is best for a patient based on the patient's daily academic and activity schedule and a child's preference for pills, liquid, or a patch. Insurance coverage can also dictate which medication is prescribed. Generic versus brand-name products can affect the out-of-pocket costs for families.

Table 1
ADHD medication guide

Medication	Available Forms	Dosage Strengths	Dosing Schedule	Approximate Duration of Action	Pattern of Release	Maximum Dose	Approved Ages	Generic Available?
Amphetamines								
Adderall (mixed amphetamine salts)	Tablet	5 mg, 7.5 mg, 10 mg, 12.5 mg, 15 mg, 20 mg, 30 mg	BID or TID	4–6 h	100% released immediately	40 mg	3 y and older	Yes
Adderall XR (mixed amphetamine salts)	Capsule (can be opened and sprinkled on soft food)	5 mg, 10 mg, 15 mg, 20 mg, 25 mg, 30 mg	Daily	8–12 h	2 equal doses, 4 h apart	30 mg	6 y and older	Yes
Vyvanse (lisdexamfetamine)	Capsule (can be opened and sprinkled on soft food or dissolved in liquid)	10 mg, 20 mg, 30 mg, 40 mg, 50 mg, 60 mg, 70 mg	Daily	10–12 h	Released continuously	70 mg	6 y and older	No
Dexedrine Spansule (dextroamphetamine sulfate)	Capsule	5 mg, 10 mg, 15 mg	Daily–BID	6–8 h	40% released immediately and 60% continuously	40 mg	6–16 y	Yes
ProCentra (dextroamphetamine)	Solution	5 mg/5 mL	BID–TID	4–6 h	100% released immediately	40 mg	3–16 y	Yes
Zenzedi (dextroamphetamine sulfate)	Tablet	2.5 mg, 5 mg, 7.5 mg, 10 mg, 15 mg, 20 mg, 30 mg	BID–TID	4–6 h	100% released immediately	40 mg	3–16 y	No
Methylphenidates								
Ritalin (methylphenidate HCl)	Tablet	5 mg, 10 mg, 20 mg	BID	2–4 h	100% released immediately	60 mg	6 y and older	Yes

Drug	Formulation	Doses	Dosing	Duration	Release	Max dose	Age	Generic
Ritalin LA (methylphenidate HCl LA)	Capsule (can be opened and sprinkled on soft food)	10 mg, 20 mg, 30 mg, 40 mg, 60 mg	Daily	6–8 h	2 equal doses, 4 h apart	60 mg	6 y and older	Yes
Ritalin SR	Tablet	20 mg	Daily	8 h	Sustained release	60 mg	6 y and older	Yes
Concerta (methylphenidate HCl ER)	Tablet (immediate-release outer coating; do not crush or chew)	18 mg, 27 mg, 36 mg, 54 mg	Daily	9–12 h	22% released immediately and 78% released continuously	72 mg	6 y and older	Yes
Focalin (dexmethylphenidate)	Tablet	2.5 mg, 5 mg, 10 mg	BID, TID	4–6 h	100% released immediately	20 mg	6 y and older	Yes
Focalin XR (Dexmethylphenidate HCl)	Capsule (can opened and sprinkled on soft food)	5 mg, 10 mg, 15 mg, 20 mg, 25 mg, 30 mg, 35 mg, 40 mg	Daily or BID	6–10 h	2 equal doses, 4 h apart	40 mg	6 y and older	Yes
Quillivant XR	Suspension (shake for 10 s before use)	25 mg/5 mL	Daily	10–12 h	Continuous release with initial onset at 45 min	60 mg	6 y and older	No
Daytrana patch (methylphenidate patch)	Transdermal patch	10 mg, 15 mg, 20 mg, 30 mg	Daily	11–12 h (remove up to 9 h after application)	Released continuously	30 mg	6–18 y old	No

(continued on next page)

Table 1
(continued)

Medication	Available Forms	Dosage Strengths	Dosing Schedule	Approximate Duration of Action	Pattern of Release	Maximum Dose	Approved Ages	Generic Available?
Aptensio XR	Capsule (can be opened and sprinkled on soft food)	10 mg, 15 mg, 20 mg, 30 mg, 40 mg, 50 mg, 60 mg	Daily	12 h	40% released within the first 2 h, reaching an initial peak at 2 h; 60% released continuously over the next 6–8 h, it troughs before it peaks again at hour 8	60 mg	6 y and older	No
Metadate CD	Capsule (can be opened and sprinkled onto soft food)	10 mg, 20 mg, 30 mg, 40 mg, 50 mg, 60 mg	Daily–BID	6–8 h	30% released immediately; 70% released continuously	60 mg	6 y and older	Yes
Methylin	Tablet	5 mg, 10 mg, 20 mg	BID–TID	3–5 h	100% released immediately	60 mg	6 y and older	Yes
Methylin chewable	Chewable tablet	2.5 mg, 5 mg, 10 mg	BID–TID	3–5 h	100% released immediately	60 mg	6 y and older	Yes
Methylin solution	Liquid	5 mg/5 mL, 10 mg/ 5 mL	BID–TID	3–5 h	10% released immediately	60 mg	6 y and older	Yes

Nonstimulants

Strattera (atomoxetine)	Capsule	10 mg, 18 mg, 25 mg, 40 mg, 60 mg, 80 mg, 100 mg	Daily	Continuous	Can take 4–8 wk to see benefits of therapy	100 mg	6 y and older	No
Kapvay (clonidine, extended release)	Tablet	0.1 mg, 0.2 mg	BID, TID, QID	Continuous	Onset of action is 1–2 wk	0.4 mg	6–17 y	Yes
Intuniv (guanfacine, extended release)	Tablet	Intuniv: 1 mg, 2 mg, 3 mg, 4 mg	Daily	Continuous	Can take 3–4 wk to see benefits of therapy	Monotherapy 6–12 y: 4 mg/d 13–17 y: 7 mg/d Adjunct therapy with stimulants: 4 mg/d	6–17 y	Yes

Medical food

Vayarin (PS, DHA, and EPA)	Capsules (can be opened and sprinkled onto soft food)	1 capsule contains: PS 75 mg, DHA 8.5 mg, and EPA 21.5 mg	2 capsules Daily	2 capsules	Can take 30–90 d to see benefits of therapy	2 capsules	Studied in children ages 6–13 y	No

Abbreviations: DHA, docosahexaenoic acid; EPA, eicosapentaenoic acid; PS, phosphatidylserine.

Dosing and titration Stimulant medications should be started at the lowest dose. They are safely titrated up to the next available dosing option every 7 to 10 days until symptoms are managed.[14] They can be titrated quickly because their effects are often seen quickly.[1] A beneficial dose is achieved when the child's behavior symptoms have improved while minimizing side effects. The provider should receive a progress report, via parental telephone call or office visit, every week while the dose is being titrated to assess the patient's behavior and any side effects.

After an effective dose has been achieved, the patient should be re-evaluated in the office by the PCP at least every 6 months to assess medication tolerance, efficacy, and growth parameters. If a patient is not successfully managed within one category of medication, the patient can change to a medication from the other category without a tapering-off period. By trying two different medication categories, this increases the overall medication response rate to 85%.[14]

Side effects All stimulant medications risk side effects, with the most common being appetite suppression and insomnia. Less common side effects include headache, abdominal pain, tics, and psychotic behavior, which are likely to resolve after several weeks of medication.[1]

Stimulant medications work by increasing noradrenaline, which increases heart rate and blood pressure. Stimulant medications come with a rare, although serious, warning that they could cause a severe cardiac event, including sudden cardiac death, in patients with a known structural heart defect or conduction disorder.[14] Individuals with a family history of sudden cardiac death are considered to be at high cardiac risk. An electrocardiogram is not required before starting stimulants unless there is a concern based on the history or physical examination. Concern about a child's cardiac risk warrants a referral to a cardiologist for clearance before initiating medication.[14]

Stimulant medications are categorized as schedule II by the Drug Enforcement Administration indicating they have a high potential for abuse, which can result in physical or psychological dependence. However, most studies indicate that individuals correctly diagnosed with ADHD and under close medical supervision are less likely to develop abusive patterns. Nevertheless, a concern remains on college campuses because students illegally buy stimulant medications to enhance academic performance or sell their medications for financial gain.[14] Clinicians either initiating or continuing treatment with stimulant medications for college students should provide education about the consequences of inappropriately using or selling these prescription medications. Students requesting refills more frequently than every month suggests abusive behavior. Students requesting refills less frequently than every month suggests poor medication compliance.

Nonstimulants

Some children are not candidates for stimulant therapy because of cardiac history, inability to manage side effects, high risk for substance abuse, or parental concern. In these scenarios, it is reasonable for the PCP to discuss nonstimulant medication options with the patient and family.

Pharmacology Atomoxetine (Strattera), a selective noradrenaline reuptake inhibitor, allows for more noradrenaline to be available for use by the neuron resulting in improved management of ADHD symptoms. Guanfacine (Intuniv), a selective α_2-adrenergic agonist antihypertensive, preferentially binds postsynaptic α_2-adrenoreceptors in the prefrontal cortex. Clonidine (Kapvay) is also an α_2-adrenergic agonist antihypertensive, and its role in the control of ADHD is not fully understood. It is presumed that postsynaptic α_2-agonist stimulation regulates subcortical activity in the prefrontal cortex to improve emotional control, working memory, attention, and behavior.[14]

Nonstimulant medications differ from stimulant medications by having a slower onset of action, a 24-hour duration, and the active ingredient accumulates in the body.[14]

Dosing and titration Nonstimulants have a slow, continuous onset of action requiring slow dose titration over the course of several weeks, and patients must titrate off of these medications.[14] Nonstimulant medications can be initiated in children 6 years and older and can be used in conjunction with stimulant medication. This is appropriate for patients requiring more symptom control but who have either reached the maximum dose for a stimulant medication or have reached their own personal stimulant dose that is limited by side effects. There is less evidence to support nonstimulant use and efficacy, and they are only one-third to one-half as effective as stimulant medications.[1,31]

Side effects The most common side effects of nonstimulant medications include headache, abdominal pain, nausea, vomiting, and somnolence, which often resolve after several weeks of consistent use. α_2-Adrenergic agonists (Intuniv, Kapvay) can decrease blood pressure and heart rate.[14]

Behavioral Therapy

Behavior therapy modifies the physical and social environment to promote behavior change. It is the primary therapy for preschool-aged children and is recommended as adjunct therapy with stimulant medications in school-aged children and adolescents.[1] Behavioral therapy is multifactorial because it involves the modification of behaviors in different settings (eg, home, school, recreational) and therefore involves the parents, teachers, and often a behavioral therapist.[5]

Evidence-based behavioral parent training is designed to enhance parental confidence in establishing boundaries in the home and enforcing positive reinforcement that improves child compliance.[1,5] Established and consistent routines help manage ADHD.

Evidence-based behavioral classroom management is meant to give teachers strategies to decrease disruptive behavior and improve work productivity and academic success.[1] Some children with ADHD can benefit from school accommodations including preferential seating, modified work assignments, test modifications (eg, allowing extended time or a different testing environment), or an individualized education plan.[1]

Outside of school, many individuals benefit from additional tutoring to improve study skills and organization. These resources may be difficult to find and are often not covered by commercial insurance. Group-based behavioral peer interventions are available to provide social-skills training and more successful peer interactions and relationships.[1]

Younger children may benefit from the use of weighted vests or fidget tools (ie, squeeze balls, taping Velcro underneath desks for the child to scratch, using a balance ball to sit on instead of a chair) to help them decrease hyperactivity and maintain focus.

Although behavioral therapy is effective at managing ADHD symptoms, it is most effective when used in conjunction with stimulant medication.[5] The success of therapy alone has been deemed equivalent to the success of nonstimulant medication alone.[5] Stimulant medications alone are more successful than therapy alone.[1]

Medical Nutrition Therapy

Well-balanced nutrition is crucial for overall childhood development and for management of any chronic condition, including ADHD. The efficacy of certain diets and supplements for patients who are trying to avoid stimulant medication or who are suboptimally controlled on medication is gaining recognition.[30] Suggested diets include lipid (fatty-acid) supplementation, immunogenic (elimination) diet, and sugar-restricted diet.

Dietary lipids

Long-chain PUFA deficiency, likely caused by either poor intake or altered metabolism, has been reported in children with ADHD.[30] Meta-analyses suggest that the combination of omega-3 and omega-6 PUFAs improves emotional and behavior problems in children with ADHD, yet is not as effective as medication monotherapy.[33,34] Based on these promising findings, a medical food in capsule form, Vayarin, is available and indicated for children ages 6 to 13 years with emotional dysregulation and hyperactivity.[31] These supplements can be trialed as monotherapy or in addition to current stimulant medications. PUFAs enhance neurotransmission, which allows an individual to use a smaller dose of stimulant medication to achieve a desirable response.[31]

Immunogenic diet

Childhood hypersensitivities (ie, eczema, gastrointestinal distress) or allergic reactions can occur with certain foods. These foods are speculated to cause a type of hypersensitive reaction in a child's brain.[35] A hypoallergenic diet eliminates foods often associated with food sensitivity, including cow's milk, cheese, wheat, egg, chocolate, nuts, and citrus fruits. The Impact of Nutrition on Children with ADHD is a randomized controlled trial that found a restricted elimination diet reduced ADHD symptoms in 64% of its pediatric subjects, whereas reintroduction of high IgG foods led to regression in behavior.[35] However, this diet is difficult to follow and results in poor compliance. Children must be monitored by a dietitian to ensure that they meet all nutritional requirements for growth.

Other dietary modifications

Society associates increased sugar and carbohydrate consumption with hyperactivity, but most controlled trials have yet to directly prove this correlation.[30] It is possible that an increased carbohydrate load can cause reactive hypoglycemia, which can result in a child's inattention and hyperactivity. Thus, it is reasonable to avoid foods with a high-glycemic index and ensure all meals and snacks include protein to avoid hypoglycemia.[30]

Mineral deficiency is correlated with worsening symptoms of ADHD. Zinc, in particular, acts as a cofactor for the metabolism of dopamine and fatty acids.[30] Iron and zinc supplementation are beneficial in the management of symptoms and enhance the effect of stimulant medication.[30]

SPECIAL CONSIDERATIONS

Given the strong inheritance of ADHD, pediatric PCPs often manage ADHD in children whose parents have ADHD. If a parent has undiagnosed or poorly managed ADHD, this increases the risk of missed appointments, delayed requests for refills, and poor time management and organization at home.

When refilling prescriptions for controlled substances, some primary care practices find it beneficial to maintain a controlled-substance log to track refill requests and to settle disputes between family members who may make multiple requests for medications because of the patient living with separated parents or caregivers.

It is not uncommon for a pediatrician to see an adolescent or young adult who presents with personal concerns that he or she has ADHD. If a young adult presents with symptoms of ADHD, and there is no previous documentation of any concerns, the clinician should suspect drug-seeking behavior and refer the patient to a specialist for an age-appropriate ADHD evaluation.

If a pediatric PCP is uncertain of an ADHD diagnosis, feels unqualified managing comorbidities, or if the child has failed several therapies because of poor compliance or significant side effects, the patient is referred to a pediatric specialist, such as a psychiatrist, neurologist, learning consultant, or behavior therapist.[1,14]

PROGNOSIS

Approximately one-third of children diagnosed with ADHD continue to struggle with their symptoms as adolescents and adults, qualifying it as a chronic medical condition.[1,4] Adolescents that discontinue treatment are significantly more likely to engage in high-risk activities.[1] Adults with undiagnosed or poorly managed ADHD have higher rates of unintentional injury, socialization and peer problems, and professional failure.[4]

However, not all individuals with ADHD require medication management for their entire life. Many can develop better organizational and task-performing skills allowing them to either decrease the dose of their medication or discontinue it entirely.

SUMMARY

As the prevalence of ADHD continues to increase because of improved awareness, more accurate diagnosis, revised DSM guidelines, and a greater number of children and adolescents with the disorder, increased numbers of parents are seeking evaluation and guidance from their PCP. Clinicians should be aware of common comorbid disorders complicating the diagnosis and management of ADHD. There are multiple medication options, behavioral therapy, and medical nutrition therapies that prove beneficial for the management of ADHD symptoms. However, if a PCP believes that a patient has complicated comorbid disorders or treatment-resistant ADHD, a referral to a psychiatrist or mental health specialist is advised. Because ADHD often persists into adulthood, the clinician must be aware of how to screen, diagnose, and manage this chronic condition so that children and adolescents have the greatest opportunity at leading a full and successful life.

REFERENCES

1. Subcommittee on Attention-Deficit/Hyperactivity Disorder, Steering Committee on Quality Improvement and Management, Wolraich M, et al. ADHD: clinical practice guideline for the diagnosis, evaluation, and treatment of attention-deficit/hyperactivity disorder in children and adolescents. Pediatrics 2011; 128:1007–22.
2. Sucksdorff M, Lehtonen L, Chudal R, et al. Preterm birth and poor fetal growth as risk factors of attention-deficit/hyperactivity disorder. Pediatrics 2015;136: e599–607.
3. American Psychiatric Association. DSM-5 attention deficit/hyperactivity disorder fact sheet. Arlington, VA: American Psychiatric Publishing; 2013. Available at: http://www.dsm5.org/documents/adhd%20fact%20sheet.pdf. Accessed December 5, 2015.

4. Visser S, Danielson M, Bitsko R, et al. Trends in the parent-report of health care provider-diagnosed and medicated attention-deficit/hyperactivity disorder: United States, 2003-2011. J Am Acad Child Adolesc Psychiatry 2014;53:34–46.

5. Fabiano G, Pelham W, Coles E, et al. A meta-analysis of behavioral treatments for attention-deficit/hyperactivity disorder. Clin Psychol Rev 2009;29:129–40.

6. Rabiner D. New diagnostic criteria for ADHD: subtle but important changes. In: Attention research update. 2013. Available at: http://www.helpforadd.com/2013/june.htm. Accessed December 17, 2015.

7. Visser S, Zablotsky B, Danielson M, et al. Diagnostic experiences of children with attention-deficit/hyperactivity disorder. Natl Health Stat Rep 2015;81:1–7.

8. Sims M, Lonigan C. Multi-method assessment of ADHD characteristics in pre-school children: relations between measures. Early Child Res Q 2012;27:329–37.

9. Willcutt E. The prevalence of DSM-IV attention-deficit/hyperactivity disorder: a meta-analytic review. Neurotherapeutics 2012;9:490–9.

10. Division of Human Development and Disability, National Center on Birth Defects and Developmental Disabilities, Center for Disease Control and Prevention. Is it ADHD? Symptoms and diagnosis. Available at: http://www.cdc.gov/ncbddd/adhd/diagnosis.html. Accessed on December 17, 2015.

11. Thomas R, Sanders S, Doust J, et al. Prevalence of attention-deficit/hyperactivity disorder: a systematic review and meta-analysis. Pediatrics 2015;135:e994–1001.

12. Boyle C, Boulet S, Schieve L, et al. Trends in the prevalence of developmental disabilities in US children, 1997-2008. Pediatrics 2011;127:1034–42.

13. Spruyt K, Gozal D. Sleep disturbances in children with attention-deficit/hyperactivity disorder. Expert Rev Neurother 2011;11:565–77.

14. Kaplan G, Newcorn J. Pharmacotherapy for child and adolescent attention-deficit hyperactivity disorder. Pediatr Clin North Am 2011;58:99–120.

15. Ahmadi N, Mohammadi M, Araghi S, et al. Neurocognitive profile of children with attention deficit hyperactivity disorders (ADHD): a comparison between subtypes. Iran J Psychiatry 2014;9:197–202.

16. Purper-Ouakil D, Ramoz N, Lepagnol-Bestel A, et al. Neurobiology of attention deficit/hyperactivity disorder. Pediatr Res 2011;69:69R–76R.

17. VanBeijsterveldt C, Middeldorp C, Landt M, et al. Influence of candidate genes on attention problems in children: a longitudinal study. Behav Genet 2011;41:155–64.

18. Elia J, Gai X, Xie H, et al. Rare structural variants found in attention-deficit hyperactivity disorder are preferentially associated with neurodevelopmental genes. Mol Psychiatry 2010;15:637–46.

19. Konikowska K, Regulska-Ilow B, Rozanska D. The influence of components of diet on the symptoms of ADHD in children. Rocz Panstw Zakl Hig 2012;63:127–34.

20. Gipson T, Lance E, Albury R, et al. Disparities in identification of comorbid diagnoses in children with ADHD. Clin Pediatr (Phila) 2015;54:376–81.

21. Conners C. DSM-5 update. In: Wiechorek D, editor. Conners. 3rd edition. (Canada): Multi-Health Systems Inc; 2014. p. 1–14.

22. Bard D, Wolraich M, Neas B, et al. The psychometric properties of the Vanderbilt Attention-Deficit Hyperactivity Disorder Diagnostic Parent Rating Scale in a community population. J Dev Behav Pediatr 2013;34:72–82.

23. Wolraich M, Bard D, Neas B, et al. The psychometric properties of the Vanderbilt Attention-Deficit Hyperactivity Disorder Diagnostic Teacher Rating Scale in a community population. J Dev Behav Pediatr 2013;34:83–93.

24. Wolraich M, Lambert W, Doffing M, et al. Psychometric properties of the Vanderbilt ADHD Diagnostic Parent Rating Scale in a referred population. J Pediatr Psychol 2003;28:559–67.
25. Bastawy M, Rabei S. The prevalence and associations of depressive episodes among children with attention-deficit hyperactive disorder (an observational cross-sectional study). Middle East Curr Psychiatry 2015;22:88–90.
26. Harstad E, Levy S, Committee on Substance Abuse. Attention-deficit/hyperactivity disorder and substance abuse. Pediatrics 2014;134:e293–301.
27. Becker S, Langberg J, Vaughn A, et al. Clinical utility of the Vanderbilt ADHD Diagnostic Parent Rating Scale comorbidity screening scales. J Dev Behav Pediatr 2012;33:221–8.
28. Sarver D, McCart M, Sheidow A, et al. ADHD and risky sexual behavior in adolescents: conduct problems and substance use as mediators of risk. J Child Psychol Psychiatry 2014;55:1345–53.
29. Trani M, Roma F, Elda A, et al. Comorbid depressive disorders in ADHD: the role of ADHD severity, subtypes and familial psychiatric disorders. Psychiatry Investig 2014;11:137–42.
30. Millichap J, Yee M. The diet factor in attention-deficit/hyperactivity disorder. Pediatrics 2012;129:330–7.
31. Rosenthal D. The potential role of lipids in ADHD. [lecture]. St Louis (Missouri): 2016.
32. Durand-Rivera A, Alatorre-Miguel E, Zambrano-Sanchez E, et al. Methylphenidate efficacy: immediate versus extended release at short term in Mexican children with ADHD assessed by conners scale and EEG. Neurol Res Int 2015; 2015:1–9.
33. Barragan E, Breuer D, Dopfner M. Efficacy and safety of omega-3/6 fatty acids, methylphenidate, and a combined treatment in children with ADHD. J Atten Disord 2014;1–9.
34. Manor I, Magen A, Keidar D, et al. The effect of phosphatidylserine containing omega3 fatty-acids on attention-deficit hyperactivity disorder symptoms in children: a double-blind placebo-controlled trial, followed by an open-label extension. Eur Psychiatry 2012;27:335–42.
35. Pelsser L, Frankena K, Toorman J, et al. Effects of a restricted elimination diet on the behavior of children with attention-deficit hyperactivity disorder (INCA study): a randomised controlled trial. Lancet 2011;377:494–503.

Printed and bound by CPI Group (UK) Ltd, Croydon, CR0 4YY

03/10/2024

01040391-0018